Tip-Edge Orthodontics

To all my National Health Service patients at Glan Clwyd Hospital, without whose cooperation this book would not have been possible

Commissioning Editor: Michael Parkinson
Project Development Manager: Lynn Watt
Project Manager: Frances Affleck
Designer: Judith Wright
Illustration Manager: Bruce Hogarth

Tip-Edge Orthodontics

Richard Parkhouse BDS Hons (Lond), FDS, DOrth, RCS (Eng)
Consultant Orthodontist, Glan Clwyd Hospital, Wales, UK

Illustration by Robert Britton

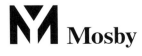 Mosby

EDINBURGH LONDON NEW YORK OXFORD PHILADELPHIA ST LOUIS SYDNEY TORONTO 2003

MOSBY An affiliate of Elsevier Science Limited
© 2003, Elsevier Science Limited. All rights reserved.

First published 2003

ISBN 0723 43228 7

British Library Cataloguing in Publication Data
A catalogue record for this book is available from the British Library

Library of Congress Cataloging in Publication Data
A catalog record for this book is available from the Library of Congress

The
publisher's
policy is to use
**paper manufactured
from sustainable forests**

Printed by the Bath Press, Bath

Preface and Acknowledgements

Tip-Edge Orthodontics has come about as a result of world-wide demand for a comprehensive textbook, outlining the use and possibilities of what is still a relatively new appliance system. It is remarkable that such a seemingly small modification to a single edgewise bracket should have such far reaching consequences and implications, overturning much established orthodontic thinking in the process. Inevitably, this means a reappraisal of the way we think, in our approach to our cases. Clearly there has been a long felt need for a definitive textbook, to stand alongside the many which have been written on edgewise and straight wire techniques, for which there is certainly no lack of guidance.

This book is therefore additional to the Tip-Edge Guide, which serves as a useful handbook, by way of introduction, coming from the birthplace of the Tip-Edge appliance and former Begg centre of excellence. It will be noted that *Tip-Edge Orthodontics* approaches Tip-Edge from a straight wire perspective, as has been long requested by those many orthodontists around the world who have participated on courses. In so doing, it fulfils my number one professional ambition, based on extensive clinical experience of Begg and straight wire techniques, by combining the very best of both worlds: the ease of differential tooth movement, with the finishing precision of a preadjusted appliance. Tip-Edge is the only bracket able to achieve this within a single archwire slot.

Inevitably, such a demanding project is not as single handed as it may appear. At Glan Clwyd Hospital, I would like to acknowledge Dr Jayne Harrison, who finally persuaded me to write the book, also Dr Joy Hickman and Dr Annabel Teague, for their proofreading and encouragement.

Pam Sheridan is surely an assistant without peer (confirmed by the many overseas visitors who have watched her at work) who has sat patiently at my side right through the years of discovery with Tip-Edge. The work of Ann Sim, hygienist, speaks for itself within these pages.

As a source of inspiration I must first mention Dr Peter Kesling, not least because he invented the bracket, and indeed his co-workers at the Kesling Rocke Orthodontic Center. These include his son Dr Chris Kesling and the late and much missed Dr Tom Rocke. It is a privilege to be able to swap ideas across the Atlantic with progressive minds, watching our baby grow and learn new tricks! Thanks are also due to TP Orthodontics Inc. for their help in providing exclusive data for the illustrations.

No book can be better than its publisher. At the outset, thank you Bill (Dr William Clark of Twin Block fame) for suggesting me to Mosby just as, unknown to you, I was about to start tapping keys, and later to Dr Colin Twelftree, for those constructive suggestions at proof stage. The energetic Michael Parkinson, as Commissioning Editor, guided me through the maze of first time authorship, while Lynn Watt, Project Development Manager, has miraculously assembled together all the pieces of a highly complex jigsaw. And not forgetting Robert Britton, artist extraordinary, who has consistently managed silk purse illustrations from my sow's ear sketches.

Closer to home, my son Paul, the engineer of the family, spent a vacation in the attic delivering the mathematical secrets locked up inside the Tip-Edge bracket, thereby greatly clarifying our understanding of what is going on in Rectangular Stage III. Lastly, and far from least, the most fortunate of authors have patient wives behind them. Rachel has been one of these, having lost me for countless hours to the computer.

I can only trust that the result will justify the efforts of many.

Richard Parkhouse

Contents

Introduction

Introduction

The Tip-Edge® (TP Orthodontics Inc., La Porte, Indiana, USA) bracket was invented by Dr Peter Kesling to introduce differential tooth movement within an edgewise based bracket system.[1-3] As its name suggests, Tip-Edge combines an initial degree of tooth tipping, which greatly facilitates tooth movement, prior to 'edgewise' precision finishing.

Based on extensive clinical experience, it is the belief of the author that Tip-Edge is the most significant innovation in fixed appliance orthodontics since the original edgewise bracket.[4,5] While essentially a 'straight-wire' appliance itself, in terms of preadjusted bracket specification and elimination of looped archwires and finishing bends, it overcomes the fundamental limitations of today's popularly accepted straight-wire systems, and opens up new horizons in fixed appliance orthodontics.

Although the title of Tip-Edge was originally coined as a nickname, it has since become adopted worldwide, in preference to the official and more formal title of Differential Straight-Arch® (TP Orthodontics Inc., La Porte, Indiana, USA) technique.

Historical perspective

Recognition is rightly given to Dr Edward Angle as the father of fixed appliance orthodontics (Fig. 1.1). The 'Edgewise' bracket, which he invented as long ago as 1925, has been the mainstay of fixed appliance practice ever since.[6] It provides the neatest way of achieving three-dimensional root control and was, in its day, years ahead of its time. Time moves on, however, and many of the intrinsic faults and limitations of edgewise based systems have since been acknowledged, but incompletely addressed.

It is little known that Angle himself appreciated that tooth movement was facilitated by allowing a tooth to tip. Previous to his edgewise bracket, he illustrated a crude piston device for retracting a canine into an extraction space, propelled by a threaded screw.[7] The attachment to the band incorporated a primitive hinge to allow distal crown tipping of the tooth being moved. Unfortunately, he had no means of subsequent root uprighting. Significantly, shortly after he conceived the edgewise bracket, he adopted his well known non-extraction treatment doctrine, to which his edgewise bracket was best

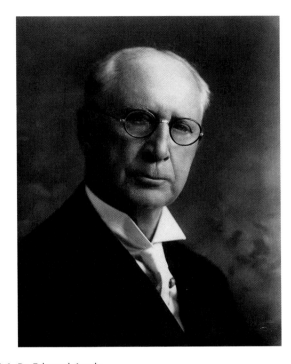

Fig. 1.1 Dr Edward Angle.

suited, although many of his results, as history shows, proved to be unstable.

While several orthodontists of the postwar period reintroduced the concept of extractions, in crowded or severe discrepancy cases, in search of greater stability, Dr Raymond Begg (Fig. 1.2) was notable in evolving a different bracket system. The resulting Begg technique marked a radical departure from conventional treatment mechanics.[8,9] In fact, the Begg bracket was itself a modification of Angle's earlier 'ribbon arch' bracket. Its adoption was designed to overcome one of the prime disadvantages inherent in all edgewise systems, which Begg had previously recognized. This is that every tooth is subject to mesio-distal bodily control from the moment of archwire engagement, thus increasing resistance to retraction.[10] By allowing teeth to tip freely during the initial stages of tooth translation, Begg introduced an entirely new sequence of tooth movement, first tipping the crowns into was able to show cases treated with a speed undreamed of with edgewise type appliances, and with a flexibility of tooth movement that enabled ultralight forces to be used. This in turn made fewer demands upon anchorage.

From the time it first appeared in the early 1960s, the Begg appliance aroused keen interest but, perhaps inevitably, was fiercely opposed by established orthodontic thinking. Much of this was no doubt provoked by the safeguarding of vested interests and the professional reputations of many. At the same time, Begg's appliance, exciting as it was, had inherent problems. Root recovery, sometimes from extreme angles, could be less than reliable, while accurate molar control and buccal segment torque were denied by the inability to use rectangular archwires.

In retrospect, Begg undoubtedly stimulated conventional edgewise thinking towards lighter forces and shorter treatment times. This has since been aided by advances in metallurgy and reduction of friction between brackets and archwires, a continuing quest which is still much in evidence today. He was also the first to demonstrate the potential of differential tooth movement.

Without question, a most notable innovation in bracket design, which continues to dominate modern orthodontics, came with the advent of the 'straight-wire' bracket system, pioneered by Dr Lawrence Andrews in the late 1970s.[11-13] This was a direct development of the edgewise design, and introduced the concept of a preadjusted appliance. By incorporating in-out adjustments and finishing angulations of tip and torque into the bracket itself, individualized finishing prescriptions for each tooth became available, based on Andrews' own research. The edgewise operator was thus relieved of the necessity of placing finishing torque into the rectangular archwires in all cases, let alone all those second order 'beautifying bends' required to achieve correct mesio-distal root angulations. Such new technology, essentially

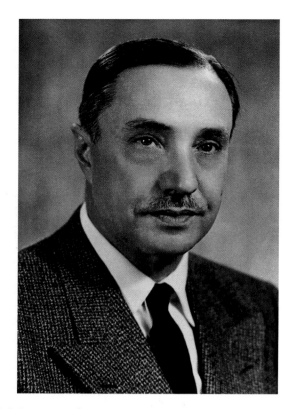

Fig. 1.2 Dr Raymond Begg.

their corrected positions before uprighting the roots as a later procedure.

It would be fair to say that Raymond Begg startled the orthodontic world in a big way. The previously unrecognized sheep farmer from Australia, who had nonetheless been a highly favoured pupil at the Angle school of orthodontics,

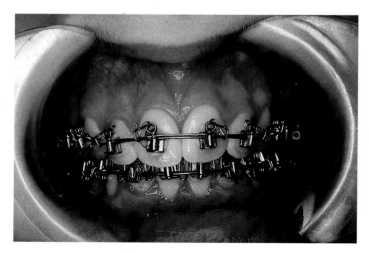
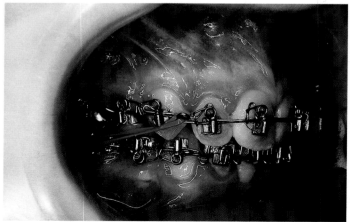

Fig. 1.3 The Begg appliance was intricate and lacked buccal segment torque. Note the auxiliary uprighting springs and spurs, correcting tip and anterior torque respectively.

simple as it was, set higher standards for case finishing, as previously defined by Andrews' six keys to normal occlusion.[14] This was further to hasten the decline of the Begg appliance, which boasted no self-limiting prescription finish and was, like edgewise, a lot more challenging to manage in terms of wire bending (Fig. 1.3).

Strictly, the term straight-wire appliance refers to the Andrews version, originally patented to the former 'A' Company, incorporating Andrews' torque in base bracket prescriptions. Subsequent alternative prescriptions appeared, notably the Roth 'modified edgewise'. Following the expiry of the patent, it was predictable that other manufacturers would follow the principle, if not the detail, giving us the plethora of so-called straight-wire brackets that we have today. The Tip-Edge bracket, at the time of writing, remains patented to TP Orthodontics.

Overcoming the limitations of conventional brackets

The undoubted popularity of straight-wire systems should not blind the free-thinking orthodontist to the many limitations that the very design of such brackets imposes, in everyday clinical use. Although simplicity of archform makes the orthodontist's life easier, and individualized bracket prescription facilitates a better detailed finish, it has long been acknowledged that moving teeth apex first generates maximum anchorage resistance. Secondly, the control of third order torque is primitive, in that torque transmitted by an active rectangular archwire inevitably provokes an unwanted reciprocal torque reaction in adjacent teeth. Finally, the torque prescription 'written in' to each bracket may not be achieved in clinical practice, due to the 10 degrees of 'torque slop' present when the commonly used .019 × .025 inch archwire is fitted within a .022 × .028 inch bracket slot.[15] Inevitably, this will result in some undertreatment, unless compensated by an exaggerated torque prescription in the bracket, or torque adjustment in the archwire.

It was primarily to address the first of the above three limitations that Dr Peter Kesling (Fig. 1.4) modified a single straight-wire bracket, to create Tip-Edge. The technique was first introduced at the Kesling-Rocke Orthodontic Center, Westville, Indiana, USA, in 1986. Although the modification to the bracket is essentially simple, confined largely to removing two diagonally opposed corners from the rectangular archwire slot, the effects are far reaching; so far reaching, in fact, that much established thinking and practice becomes challenged as obsolete by the evidence of clinical results, and particularly by the relative ease with which these can be obtained.

None of the foregoing is intended to deny the continuing excellence of the straight-wire appliance in terms of simple

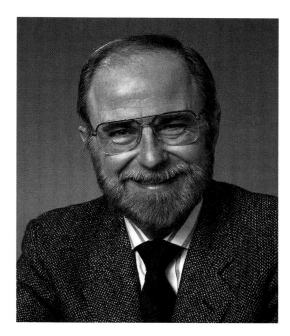

Fig. 1.4 Dr Peter Kesling.

alignment, which was, after all, the purpose for which Angle designed his edgewise bracket in the first place. Indeed, in such cases, Tip-Edge confers little or no advantage. However, the more difficult the case in terms of tooth movement, whether with extractions or non-extraction, the greater the benefit of Tip-Edge becomes. Why is this? Essentially, differential tooth movement makes the translation of teeth into their finishing positions so much easier, employing only very light forces. As will be demonstrated in later chapters, reduction of large overjets and the attainment of Class I buccal segment occlusions is greatly simplified, consuming little anchorage, while the correction of overjets and increased overbites early in treatment contributes to shorter overall treatment times.[16,17]

While it is commonly believed that the superior treatment ability of Tip-Edge is shown most convincingly in Class II division 1 and Class II division 2 cases, its flexibility of treatment is appropriate to all malocclusion types. A particular advantage, whatever the case under treatment, is that its root uprighting capability, in the rectangular wire phase, is virtually 'maintenance free'. Essentially this means that the latter half of treatment consists mainly of inspections, rather than archwire checks, entailing a considerable saving in clinical time. Furthermore, Tip-Edge is capable of delivering its finishing prescription more accurately than conventional brackets, without the need for torque adjustment in the archwire. This is because, at the conclusion of treatment, zero tolerance is achieved between bracket and rectangular archwire.

REFERENCES

1. Kesling PC. Expanding the horizons of the edgewise arch wire slot. American Journal of Orthodontics 1988; 94: 26–37.

2. Kesling PC. Differential tooth movement Tip-Edge concept and the differential straight-arch technique. Journal of Indian Orthodontics 1988; 19: 31–35.

3. Kesling PC. Dynamics of the Tip-Edge bracket. American Journal of Orthodontics 1989; 96: 16–28.

4. Parkhouse RC. New thinking with Tip-Edge. Kieferorthop 1995; 9: 137–142.

5. Parkhouse RC. JIOS-Interviews: Dr Richard Parkhouse on Tip-Edge. Journal of Indian Orthodontic Society 1992; 23: 67–73.

6. Angle EH. The latest and best in orthodontic mechanism. Dental Cosmos 1929; 71: 164–174, 260–270, 409–421.

7. Angle EH. Treatment of malocclusion of the teeth, 7th edn. Philadelphia, The SS White Dental Manufacturing Company, 1907.

8. Begg PR. Light arch wire technique employing the principles of differential force. American Journal of Orthodontics 1961; 47: 30–48.

9. Begg PR. Choice of bracket for the light wire technique. Begg Journal of Orthodontic Theory and Treatment 1962; 1: 11–17.

10. Begg PR. Differential force in orthodontic treatment. American Journal of Orthodontics 1956; 42: 481–510.

11. Andrews LF. The straight-wire appliance, origin, controversy, commentary. Journal of Clinical Orthodontics 1976; 10: 99–114.

12. Andrews LF. The straight-wire appliance. Explained and compared. Journal of Clinical Orthodontics 1976; 10: 174–195.

13. Andrews LF. The straight-wire appliance. British Journal of Orthodontics 1979; 6: 124–143.

14. Andrews LF. The six keys to normal occlusion. American Journal of Orthodontics 1972; 62: 296–309.

15. McLaughlin RP, Bennett JC, Trevisi HJ. Systemized orthodontic treatment mechanics, 2001. London: Mosby.

16. Galicia-Ramos GA, Killiany DM, Kesling PC. A comparison of standard edgewise, preadjusted edgewise, and tip-edge in Class II extraction treatment. Journal of Clinical Orthodontics 2001; 35: 145–153.

17. Kesling PC, Rocke RT, Kesling CK. Treatment with Tip-Edge brackets and differential tooth movement. American Journal of Orthodontics and Dentofacial Orthopaedics 1991; 99: 387–402.

Differential tooth movement

Differential tooth movement

It is customary, in contemporary fixed appliance orthodontics, to work towards finishing angulations from the outset of treatment. This is because edgewise derived brackets, in common use today, dictate this upon the orthodontist by exerting mesio-distal second order root forces from the time of first engagement with an archwire. The very design of such a bracket therefore imposes a treatment regimen of bodily movement (Fig. 2.1) and with it, over many years, has grown the widespread assumption that this is the way teeth require to be moved.

Yet it has long been recognized, even in classical edgewise therapy, that positioning a root apex toward the direction of pull will generate resistance to tooth movement in response to that force. It was for this reason that Dr Charles Tweed developed the concept of 'anchorage preparation', moving his apices mesially in the mandibular buccal segments by means of second order bends, so as to increase anchorage resistance to Class II elastic traction. Evidently, he used the analogy of tent pegs to illustrate his concept, whereby such pegs are driven into the ground at an angle, in order to resist the pull

of the guy rope (RT Williams, personal communication). Yet today, it seems to have become accepted practice to retract teeth apex first. This is particularly so with straight-wire brackets, which prescribe a distal root angulation to canines during retraction; similarly during overjet reduction, using rectangular archwires in pretorqued incisor brackets will induce palatal root torque which, by the simple laws of physics, will increase resistance to the desired palatal crown movement.

By complete contrast, a bracket designed for differential tooth movement will not impart root-angulating forces when an archwire is engaged. Instead, the crown will be able to tip in the direction of desired tooth movement, essentially leaving the root apex to trail behind (Fig. 2.2). Obviously, such simple free tipping requires far less force and anchorage than moving the same tooth bodily, although this would in itself amount to incomplete treatment. However, it makes initial decrowding and reduction of big overjets dramatically easy, as well as rapid, together with the attainment of a Class I buccal segment occlusion. Both are achieved early in

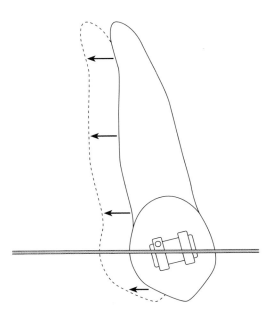

Fig. 2.1 Bodily movement during retraction with an edgewise derived bracket.

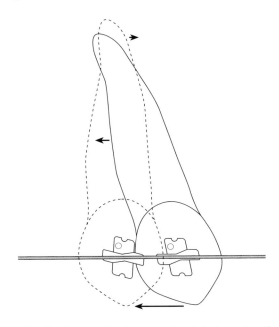

Fig. 2.2 Initial distal crown tipping permitted during retraction with a Tip-Edge bracket.

treatment. This in turn lends stability to the subsequent root uprighting process, both by establishing a strong interdigitation and by bringing the labial segments within the safety of normal lip control, as opposed to the adverse influences of lip trapping.

Of course, this constitutes only half the treatment and the root uprighting, necessary to produce finishing root angulations, may occupy the latter half of the total treatment time (Fig. 2.3). Inevitably, this has anchorage consequences, which will be discussed in Chapter 14. However, it is a striking feature of differential tooth movement that total anchorage requirements, and duration of treatment, seem significantly less than with straight-wire or edgewise systems, particularly in difficult cases.[1,2] No doubt protagonists for the conventional will wish to challenge this claim, on grounds of lack of scientific evidence; indeed it would be difficult to measure anchorage objectively. Nevertheless, on clinical evidence, it is unarguable.

Why this should be so remains unexplained. Following treatment of any malocclusion, the ideal finish should be the same, whether treated by bodily movement or by differential tooth movement (crown tipping followed by root uprighting); either way, the total change, in terms of individual tooth movement, will be identical. Therefore, one might logically expect the total anchorage demands to be the same in both cases, which they evidently are not.

There is also the clinically observed phenomenon whereby teeth seem to intrude more readily if the roots are allowed angular freedom during the process. The relevance of canine inclination to overbite reduction accounts

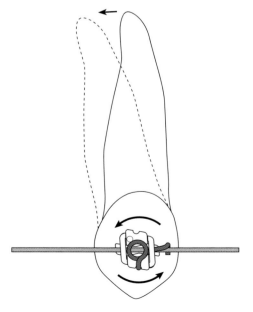

Fig. 2.3 Subsequent root uprighting of a tooth previously tipped during retraction.

for much of this, as will be understood from the next chapter.

Variable anchorage

With differential tooth movement, root torque to the bracketed teeth is imparted by the placement of auxiliary springs, rather than automatically from first archwire engagement. Although this constitutes an additional clinical procedure, the fact that the orthodontist now has the choice of which roots to control and when, introduces the concept of variable anchorage control. This is an option which is not possible with conventional brackets, without resort to more complicated add-ons such as lingual arches, headgears or other anchorage reinforcement. Obviously, during the finishing phase of treatment, all root angulations must be corrected, but during the preceding stages, variable anchorage constitutes an invaluable 'steerage mechanism' towards the control of profile and, as we shall see later, correction of centrelines.

As an example, let us consider a lower canine in an extraction case, in which the labial segment has been aligned. When closing the residual extraction space with intramandibular forces, the orthodontist can choose between retraction or protraction. If lingual movement of the labial segment is required, this will readily be achieved simply by pitting bodily movement of the first molars against the lower anteriors, all of which are free to tip, the incisors lingually and the canines distally (Fig. 2.4). Alternatively, if the labial segment position is satisfactory, anterior anchorage can be increased very easily by adding auxiliary springs to the canines (Fig. 2.5). These will induce a distal root force to both lower canines, which will buttress the anterior segment against retroclination, so long as the space-closing forces are kept light. The result will therefore be protraction. Auxiliary springs used in this way are known as 'brakes'. As will be seen in Chapter 10, it is also possible to use springs in an opposite mode to induce distal crown movement, a technique known as 'power tipping'.

Light forces

It is fundamental to differential tooth movement that all forces should be light. For example, a mere 50 grams of intermaxillary elastic force, bilaterally, will be found quite sufficient for the reduction of even large overjets. Heavier forces, as will be familiar to users of edgewise type appliances, are unnecessary and can be harmful. Not only will posterior anchorage be strained, but the periodontal ligament could be put at risk. This is because differential tooth movement naturally implies a differential periodontal response. Compared with moving a tooth bodily, when the rate of periodontal response will theoretically be uniform down the

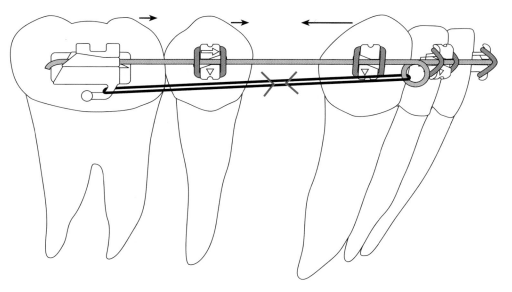

Fig. 2.4 Mechanics of retraction. Six anterior units, free to tip, offer little anchorage resistance when pitted against bodily control of the first molars. The response to intramaxillary space closing forces will therefore be anterior retraction, with minimal loss of anchorage from the molars.

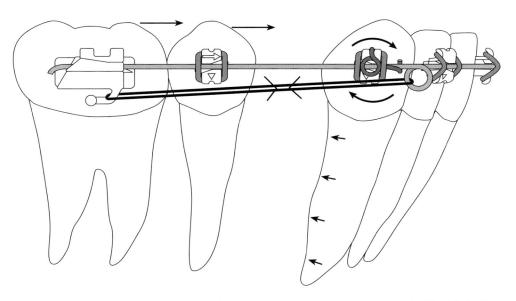

Fig. 2.5 Mechanics of protraction. A similar set-up to that in Figure 2.4, but with Side-Winder™ brakes to canines. These impart root resistance, hence increased anchorage resistance anteriorly. The response to the same space-closing forces will now be protraction of the molars.

length of the root (assuming absolute archwire rigidity), tipping a tooth will induce more root movement towards the gingival, diminishing towards the apex, which may even show slight reverse movement. The forces are therefore less evenly dissipated along the root. With light forces, this will not present problems.

It is well recognized that root resorption can occur, particularly in susceptible individuals, whatever appliance is used. However, research studies have failed to implicate differential tooth movement and the reader is referred to Beck and Harris, who list a comprehensive bibliography.[3] It should also be noted that their particular study involved the Begg appliance, which allowed angles of tip considerably greater than Tip-Edge.

Root uprighting

Before exploring differential tooth movement in detail with Tip-Edge, it is necessary to dispel one further myth. It is

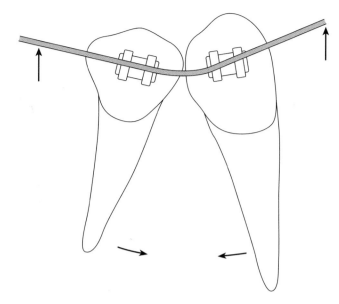

Fig. 2.6 Correcting tipped teeth with conventional brackets induces vertical archwire deflections.

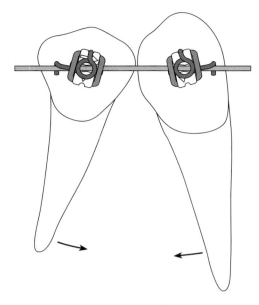

Fig. 2.7 Uprighting teeth with light auxiliary springs causes no vertical deflection of a heavy (passive) archwire.

popularly believed among students of modern orthodontics that it is 'wrong' to allow teeth to tip during treatment. This is despite the fact that a number of edgewise and straight-wire clinicians have attempted to introduce a modicum of tipping into an otherwise rigid system, in search of greater flexibility and ease of movement, by use of undersized or flexible archwires, narrow brackets or segmental arches. However, such methods are only able to exploit the advantages of differential tooth movement to a minimal extent.

Certainly, no user of conventional brackets would be able to entertain angles of tip that can be accommodated by Tip-Edge. This is hardly surprising, for the simple reason that edgewise and straight-wire brackets offer very poor recovery from tipped angulations. As can be seen (Fig. 2.6), correction of mesio-distal crown tip by engaging the brackets with an

active archwire provokes major vertical consequences, with extrusion of adjacent teeth. While addition of reciprocal gingival power arms may facilitate the uprighting process, the vertical archwire deflections remain. With Tip-Edge, however, recovery is by the light and progressive action of auxiliary springs, while vertical arch stability is maintained by a relatively heavy (but passive) archwire (Fig. 2.7).

Likewise, correction of palatally tipped incisors by means of an actively torqued rectangular archwire imposes unwanted reciprocal torque reactions on neighbouring teeth, or even the buccal segments, as mentioned in the previous chapter. In this, Tip-Edge innovates by using rectangular wire as a passive platform, to which teeth are torqued entirely individually, again by means of auxiliaries, and without torque disturbance to adjacent teeth.[4]

REFERENCES

1. Kesling CK. Differential anchorage and the Edgewise appliance. Journal of Clinical Orthodontics 1994; 28: 84–92.
2. Kesling CK. The Tip-Edge concept: eliminating unnecessary anchorage strain. Journal of Clinical Orthodontics 1992; 26: 165–178.
3. Beck NB, Harris EF. Apical root resorption in orthodontically treated subjects: analysis of edgewise and light wire mechanics. American Journal of Orthodontics and Dentofacial Orthopaedics 1994; 105: 350–361.
4. Parkhouse RC. Rectangular wire and third order torque: a new perspective. American Journal of Orthodontics 1998; 113: 421–430.

Dynamics of Tip-Edge

Dynamics of Tip-Edge

The Rx-1 bracket

The best inventions are frequently the simplest. The prototype Tip-Edge brackets were derived from a single .022 inch straight-wire bracket merely by cutting away two diametrically opposed corners from the archwire slot (Fig. 3.1), thereby allowing differential tooth movement.[1] Each bracket is thus enabled to tip in a predetermined direction, whereas with a full thickness archwire in place, it will resist tipping in the reverse direction. The desired direction of tipping, in routine orthodontic cases, is easy to predict: in general, distal crown tipping is the way the bracketed teeth will naturally want to incline, the exception being the second premolars in first premolar extraction cases, which will require to tip mesially into the extraction spaces. There are other rare exceptions to this rule, such as where anterior teeth are missing when, unless restoring the spaces, a canine may need to be moved mesially, sometimes requiring a contralateral bracket.

The Tip-Edge bracket (Fig. 3.2) contains many features already familiar to the edgewise or straight-wire operator, including conventional tie wings, which accept standard elastomeric ligatures. Likewise, bracket identification is by small circular markers at the disto-gingival tie wings of the maxillary anterior brackets, and similarly placed triangular markings for the mandibular anteriors. (The orientation of premolar brackets depends on the desired direction of tipping and is dealt with in Chapter 6.)

In common with some current straight-wire brackets, a vertical slot is incorporated lingual to the main archwire slot, which accommodates a range of possible auxiliaries. The dimension of the vertical auxiliary slot is .020 inches square, with a rounded 'funnel shaped' entry to facilitate insertion (Fig. 3.3). The strangely shaped inner surface to the main

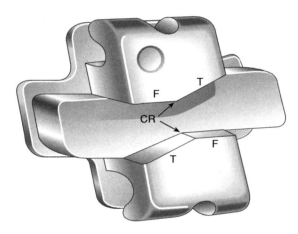

Fig. 3.2 Tip-Edge Rx-1 bracket. CR = central ridge, T = tip-limiting surfaces, F = finishing surfaces.

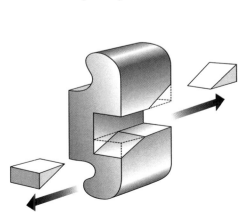

Fig. 3.1 Single straight-wire bracket minus two diametrically opposed wedges = Tip-Edge!

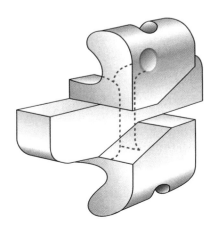

Fig. 3.3 The vertical slot for auxiliaries has a rounded entry.

archwire slot, due to the lateral extensions, is sometimes referred to as a 'propeller slot'. This preserves rotational control throughout the range of tip permitted by the bracket, without detriment to aesthetics, since it is concealed beneath the archwire itself.

The 'cut out surfaces' of the archwire slot form the 'tip-limiting surfaces', which restrict the degree of tipping permitted during tooth translation. The intact surfaces are therefore the 'finishing surfaces', containing the individualized finishing prescription for each tooth. The point at which the tip limiting and finishing surfaces meet constitutes the central ridge; the opposing central ridges provide vertical control until final finishing and are also the points at which torque is imparted, under the influence of auxiliary springs, during the final rectangular wire phase.

The basic sequence of Tip-Edge treatment is therefore illustrated, showing an upper right canine from its starting position (Fig. 3.4A). During the initial decrowding or overjet reduction, the crown will tip distally into a corrected Class I relationship. Since no root angulating forces are imparted, anchorage will be extremely light during this stage. In an extreme case, the amount of distal crown tip will be limited by the tip-limiting surface (Fig. 3.4B), so that excessive tipping is prevented. In the Rx-1 bracket, the tip-limiting surfaces are angled 25 degrees to the horizontal on canines, 20 degrees on all other bracketed teeth, although in clinical practice such maximum angles of tip will rarely be encountered.

Once all crowns are correctly placed, a Side-Winder auxiliary spring is added (Fig. 3.4C). This will distalize the root to its prescribed angulation against a passive rectangular archwire, at which point the action of the spring will become self-limited by the approximation of the finishing surfaces above and below the archwire (Fig. 3.4D).

The preadjusted finishing prescription contained within the Rx-1 bracket system is identical in principle to today's straight-wire systems, with tip in the face, torque in the base. The values (Table 3.1) are particular to Tip-Edge, but alongside various prescriptions in common use today, they compare most closely to Roth specification.

It should be mentioned that TP Orthodontics also market a Twin version of the Tip-Edge bracket in both .018 and .022 inch formats, sometimes known as the 'Freedom' bracket, perhaps in an attempt to identify more closely with conventional brackets. In the author's opinion, neither can be recommended. Apart from the obvious aesthetic disadvantages, the extra bulk of such brackets can predispose to occlusal interferences. Furthermore the internal geometry has been modified, compared with the Rx-1 bracket, placing the Side-Winder spring at some mechanical disadvantage when deriving torque against rectangular wire. Finally, it has to be said that the last thing that Tip-Edge needs is an '018' system! Light forces and flexibility are already inherent in the use of auxiliary springs. It is therefore undesirable to sacrifice overall control by introducing unwanted flexibility in the

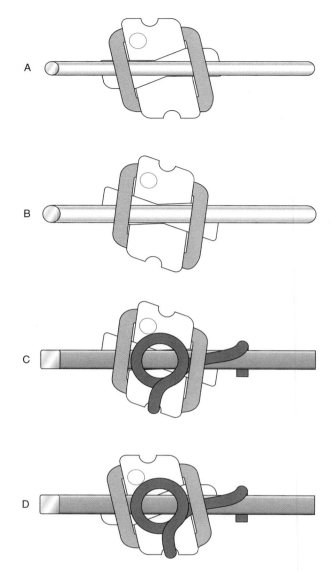

Fig. 3.4 The sequence of differential tooth movement: (A) maxillary right canine at start of Stage I. (B) By end of Stage II, following retraction, the crown will have tipped distally. (C) using a rectangular Stage III archwire, a counter-clockwise Side-Winder spring will commence root uprighting. (D) Because the archwire is rectangular, torque will be achieved automatically with tip correction, until the bracket prescription is expressed. The action is self-limiting.

passive base archwires, particularly during root uprighting, when the Side-Winders will be further handicapped by working against a narrower torquing platform.

A dynamic slot

A curious feature of the bracket design, which is unique to Tip-Edge, is that the archwire slot increases its vertical dimension as the tooth tips. As can be seen (Fig. 3.5), tipping

Table 3.1   Rx-I—Single wing Tip-Edge bracket .022 inch archwire slot angulations

	Maximum crown tip during translation	Final crown tip	Final root torque
Maxillary			
Central incisor	20° distal	5°	12°
Lateral incisor	20° distal	9°	8°
Canine	25° distal	11°	–4°
First premolar	20° distal or mesial	0°	–7°
Second premolar	20° distal or mesial	0°	–7°
Mandibular			
Central incisor	20° distal	2°	–1°
Lateral incisor	20° distal	2°	–1°
Canine	25° distal	5°	–11°
First premolar	20° distal or mesial	0°	–20°
Second premolar	20° distal or mesial	0°	–20°

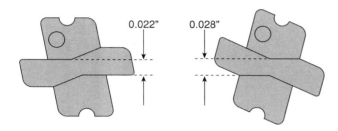

Fig. 3.5 The 'dynamic' Tip-Edge archwire slot increases its vertical archwire space as the tooth tips during initial translation.

of the tooth crown, during initial translation, alters the axial inclination between bracket and archwire, progressively increasing the vertical space available for the archwire from .022 to a maximum of .028 inches. How does this happen? The explanation lies in the geometry of the bracket, in which the mesio-distal width of the tip-limiting surfaces slightly exceeds the width of the finishing surfaces. The finishing surfaces therefore extend less that halfway across the face of the bracket, and are at no point directly opposed. Therefore the central ridges, being slightly offset either side of the mid-point, 'open up' the vertical dimension as the bracket tilts.

This feature has considerable clinical significance. Levelling and aligning is greatly assisted, so much so that it is possible to step up from a .016 to a .022 inches stainless archwire in a single move. In this context, it should also be mentioned that interbracket distance is far greater than with any conventional twin type bracket as, with Tip-Edge, the interbracket span is effectively the distance between the central ridges. No less significant, and relevant to later chapters, the dynamic slot makes possible an entirely new means of torque delivery, when the vertical slot dimension is closed down by an auxiliary spring, against a rectangular archwire, to produce a three-dimensional precision finish.

Vertical reactions during retraction

Particularly when canines are retracted along an archwire, using full arch mechanics with edgewise or straight-wire brackets, there is a well recognized tendency to produce adverse vertical reactions. This is because such brackets compel the tooth being retracted to move bodily (Fig. 3.6). By the simple laws of physics, the resistance offered by the root will tend to rotate the crown distally, causing some flexion in the archwire. This will in turn tend to extrude the labial segment and intrude the buccal segments, hence the so-called 'roller coaster' effect.

Because differential tooth movement leaves the apex behind, crown retraction carries no vertical consequences (Fig. 3.7), so that vertical 'round tripping' of the anteriors is avoided. There must, of course, be vertical implications later along the line, when the roots are eventually uprighted; however, by this stage the patient will be in heavy archwires and protected by an already established interarch relationship.

Frictional resistance

In modern orthodontics, means are constantly being sought to reduce friction between brackets and archwire. Differential tooth movement largely sidesteps this problem, for reasons stemming from the previous paragraph. The apical resistance generated when retracting a tooth bodily is the main culprit in causing binding between bracket and archwire. By contrast, leaving the apex behind will eliminate binding, particularly with a bracket that increases its vertical slot space as it retracts. When the root finally needs uprighting, the crown will already have been corrected and is, therefore, stationary relative to the archwire.

An additional point to be considered must be friction due to the elastomeric modules. However, it should be noted that, with free-sliding mechanics, the archwire will itself move distally with the teeth being retracted, particularly during overjet reduction. Interestingly, self-locking Tip-Edge brackets

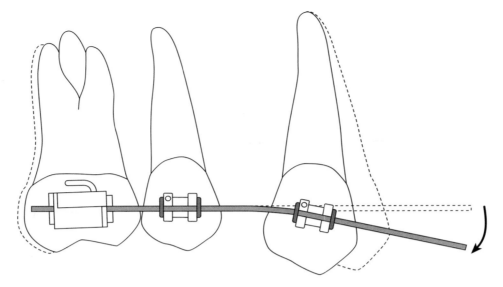

Fig. 3.6 Retraction of a canine with conventional brackets has vertical consequences, which may extrude the incisor segment.

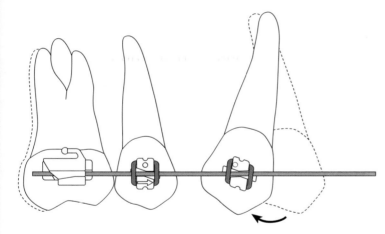

Fig. 3.7 Retraction with Tip-Edge has no extrusive effect.

have been tried clinically and found to confer little benefit compared with straight wire. A likely reason is that the large interbracket span and increased vertical space within the Rx-1 slot are helpful in allowing vertical play within each bracket, so that unresolved stresses between archwire and bracket will be more readily relieved by forces of mastication.

Bite opening

Early bite opening is one of the key reasons why differential tooth movement so frequently demonstrates a reduction in treatment times, particularly in deep bite cases. Edgewise type brackets, used with full archwires, are unable to intrude incisor segments until the canine root angulations are

corrected, which in turn delays overjet reduction. A straight-wire bracket exacerbates this problem (Fig. 3.8, see p. 19) by prescribing a greater distal root inclination, which requires to be achieved clinically before the curve of Spee can be levelled. A segmental arch approach can overcome this problem, but at the expense of added complexity.[2,3] Segmental arches are never required with Tip-Edge and, as will be seen in the clinical cases illustrated, overbite reduction can take place from the outset, irrespective of canine angulation (Fig. 3.9, see p. 19).

Molar tubes

In the interests of combining the advantages of both straight-wire and Begg modes of treatment, Tip-Edge employs double buccal tubes. These comprise a normally sited preadjusted straight-wire rectangular tube of .022 × .028 inches, which is convertible, and a gingivally placed round tube of .036 inch internal diameter (Fig. 3.10, see p. 20). The rectangular tubes are of Easy-Out® (TP Orthodontics Inc., La Porte, Indiana, USA) design, with the posterior inner lumen slightly flared towards the occlusal. This facilitates archwire removal when a cinch back has been used.

As will be seen later, use of the round tubes is confined to bite opening in the initial stages of treatment in deep bite cases. Thereafter, all space closure and root uprighting is carried out in the rectangular tubes. This naturally raises the question as to how necessary the round tubes really are. The answer to this will become apparent in the chapters on Stage I, in that the round tubes do offer significant advantages when deriving molar anchorage and bite opening from 'anchor bends', during

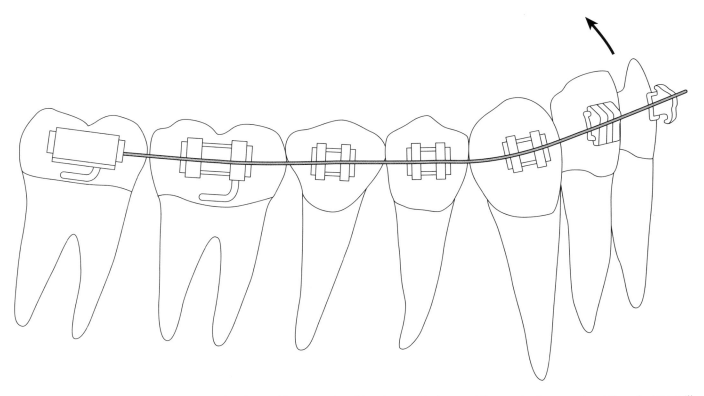

Fig. 3.8 A mesial canine apex has vertical implications with conventional brackets: anterior overbite may be increased and its reduction will be delayed until the canine angulation is corrected.

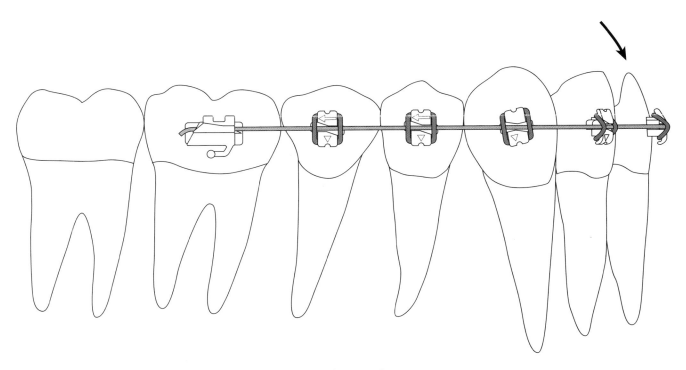

Fig. 3.9 With Tip-Edge, adverse canine angulation does not impede bite opening.

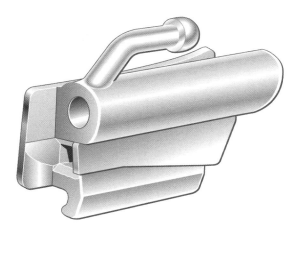

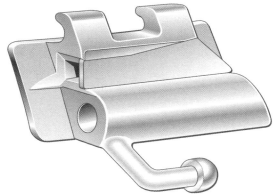

Fig. 3.10 Convertible molar tubes of Easy-Out design.

which their more gingival position gives better protection from occlusal trauma. In addition, the increased length of the round tubes makes more efficient use of the anchorage bend in terms of bite opening, as well as reducing the friction arising from it.

It will be seen that triple upper molar tubes are used in the cases illustrated in this book. In fact, headgear is very seldom required with the Tip-Edge appliance, compared with straight wire, and the presence of headgear tubes in all cases is simply the result of departmental standardization of bands. In this respect, it is worth mentioning that triple upper and double lower molar tubes will allow both straight-wire and Tip-Edge techniques to be practised side by side with a single inventory of prewelded bands.

REFERENCES

1. Kesling PC. Tip-Edge Guide and the Differential Straight-arch Technique, 4th edn. Two Swan Advertising, 2000.
2. Burstone CJ. Deep overbite correction by intrusion. American Journal of Orthodontics 1977; 72: 1–22.
3. Ricketts RM. Development of the utility arch. Foundation for Orthodontic Research Newsletter 1974; 5: 37–40.

Auxiliaries

Auxiliaries

Tip-Edge can be used with a host of different auxiliaries. Many of these are Begg derived and designed for orthodontists unfamiliar with rectangular wire. (For information on the Deep Groove torque bar system, individual root torquing auxiliary and torquing spurs, the reader is referred to the 'Tip-Edge Guide'.[1]) However, used in conjunction with rectangular wire, the Side-Winder answers all torquing requirements and is therefore the only 'root moving' spring necessary. The orthodontist's armoury of auxiliaries is therefore reduced to three: the Side-Winder, Power Pin™ (a traction hook) and the occasionally useful Rotating Spring.

The Side-Winder

This is the everyday 'workhorse' among Tip-Edge auxiliaries (Fig. 4.1). It generates mesio-distal root movement and, when used in conjunction with rectangular archwires, produces torque correction as well. It is made in .014 inch high tensile stainless steel.

So called because it carries its coils alongside the archwire, over the bracket face, the Side-Winder is a significant improvement over the former Begg type uprighting spring, which carried its coils gingivally. Because the coils of the Side-Winder are concentric with the point of second order rotation of the bracket, its action is mechanically more efficient, and its hook no longer travels noticeably along the archwire as the tooth uprights. It is also more aesthetic and easier for the patient to keep clean, although it does inevitably add to the labial profile of the bracket.

The Side-Winder has undergone considerable development since it was first introduced. Original versions were retained in the vertical slots by bending the protruding gingival tails 90 degrees, which made them fiddlesome to remove. It was subsequently realized that the spring pressure of the activated arm reciprocally keeps the tail of the spring securely seated up the vertical slot, so that the long tails were deleted. However, by far the most significant improvement has come with the so-called 'Invisible Side-Winder' (Fig. 4.2).

This is not strictly invisible, of course, although aesthetics are improved by the fact that the wire of the spring overlays the bracket and archwire so that, unless using ceramic brackets, the show of metal is scarcely increased. Perhaps of greater importance, it has several functional advantages, all of

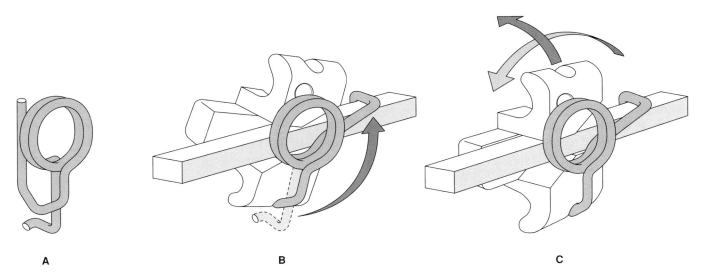

A   **B**   **C**

Fig. 4.1 A Side-Winder (A), inserted from the occlusal (upper right central) incisor (B). When the arm is hooked over the archwire (C), tip correction (light arrow) and torque correction (dark arrow) will result. The elastomeric module has been omitted in the interest of clarity.

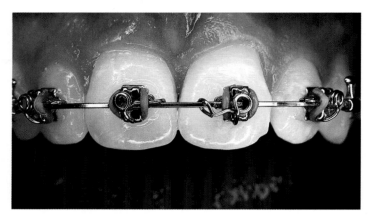

Fig. 4.2 The Invisible Side-Winder (left), compared with its predecessor (right). Note that the Invisible spring is retained by the elastomeric module, and must therefore be fitted before the module is placed.

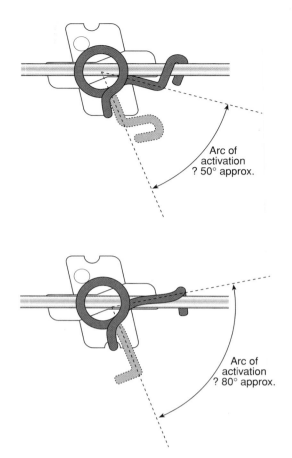

Fig. 4.3 The bulky hook of earlier Side-Winders reduced the arc of activation (above), compared with the latest Invisible design (below).

which render previous designs obsolete. Firstly, it is retained in position by the elastomeric module, in addition to its own spring pressure. This also enables the modules to be changed if necessary, during the root uprighting process, without removing the springs. Secondly, because the bulky hook has been eliminated, the spring arm has a wider range of activation than was previously possible (Fig. 4.3). While the extra power of the spring is an advantage, particularly on incisors, when delivering the final torque prescription, it is unnecessarily strong for simple second order tipping movements. Some reduction of activation on canines and premolars may frequently be indicated, therefore, in order not to strain anchorage during the uprighting phase.

Side-Winders come in clockwise and counter-clockwise formats, the one a mirror image of the other (Fig. 4.4). Selection of the correct spring for each tooth is a simple matter, according to the direction of second order correction required, as seen from the labial. Hence an upper right canine requiring distal root correction will need a counter-clockwise spring, while uprighting a lower right canine root distally will require a clockwise rotation, and so forth. It should be noted here that the selection of Side-Winders is made solely on second order considerations, irrespective of whatever torque may be required. The torque, although generated by the auxiliary, is delivered according to the setting of the rectangular archwire, as will be seen in Chapter 14 on Stage III.

Side-Winder springs should always be inserted from the occlusal and never gingivally. Admittedly the action of the spring will be the same either way, so that on a typodont the direction of insertion might seem irrelevant. But typodonts don't eat! In the mouth, the forces of mastication coming occlusally will be deflected harmlessly off the coils of a correctly inserted spring, keeping these in close proximity to the bracket face. However, if the spring is inserted upside-down, from the gingival, the occlusal forces will impact beneath the coils and

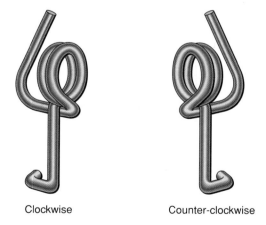

Clockwise   Counter-clockwise

Fig. 4.4 Clockwise and counter-clockwise Side-Winders.

distort them labially, away from the bracket. This spoils the action of the spring as well as causing discomfort.

The direction of action of each spring can easily be 'read' in the mouth by the clinician, according to the direction of the

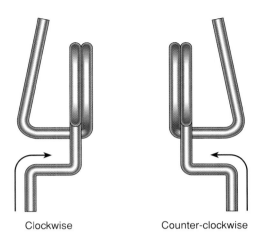

Clockwise   Counter-clockwise

Fig. 4.5 Identifying a Side-Winder: as seen, hook facing, in which direction does the wire turn away from its cut end? If clockwise, it is a clockwise spring and vice-versa.

spring arm. Since each spring is inserted occlusally, the spring arm points in the direction towards which the occlusal tip will rotate. Almost invariably, therefore, Side-Winder spring arms point mesially, the main exception being the second premolar when the first premolar has been extracted: here the second premolar root will need mesial uprighting into the extraction site. This equates to a distal rotation of its occlusal tip. Therefore, the spring arm will point to the distal (see Fig. 17.5).

It is also useful for the orthodontist to know how to 'read' Side-Winders out of the mouth, such as when replacing springs that have been removed. Confusion can easily be prevented by a simple method of recognition: holding the spring in a plier, hook facing the operator, in which direction does the hook curve? Starting from its free end, if the hook curves away in a clockwise direction, it is a clockwise spring, and vice-versa (Fig. 4.5).

As with any auxiliary spring, Side-Winders should only be used with stainless steel arches, since nickel-titanium or multistrand archwires are insufficiently stiff to resist the vertical deflections arising from the active arms of the springs.

Finally, it needs to be said that steel ligature ties and Side-Winders do not mix. The reason is that stainless steel is insufficiently elastic to allow the bracket to rotate relative to the archwire, as is necessary for the correction of both tip and torque. A wire ligature will therefore restrict the action of the spring. Consequently, Side-Winders must only be used in conjunction with elastomeric ligatures, which can readily change shape to accommodate to angular changes as they occur.

Power Pin

This is a traction hook that can be fitted in the vertical slot (Fig. 4.6). Made of soft stainless steel, it will normally be inserted from the gingival, and is retained in the slot by

bending the occlusally projecting tail 90 degrees (Fig. 4.7). Strictly, this bend should be made in the opposite direction to the elastic pull, since this avoids the possibility of a slackly turned pin doing a 'U-turn' and being pulled out of the slot by the elastic.

It can be seen in side view that the head of the Power Pin is angled relative to the shaft (Fig. 4.8). The pin should therefore be inserted with the head inclining away from the tooth or gingival margin, rather than towards it. Once fitted, the Power Pin can be left in place for as long as required; it does not interfere with arch checks. When finished with, its removal is easy, by straightening the tail and cutting it with ligature cutters.

Power Pins are most commonly used as hooks for seating elastics in the final treatment visits. However, they are also useful on the few occasions when an individual tooth requires

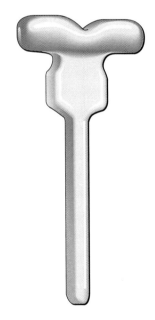

Fig. 4.6 A Power Pin.

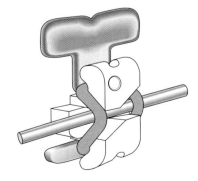

Fig. 4.7 A Power Pin is retained in the vertical slot by bending the tail 90 degrees.

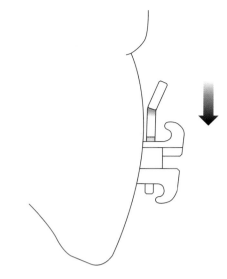

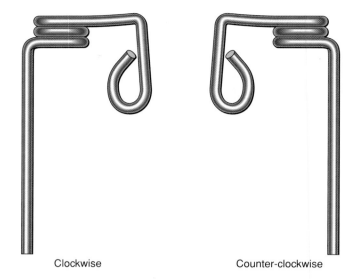

Clockwise   Counter-clockwise

Fig. 4.8 Power Pin in side view. Note that the head is angled from the shaft, and should be fitted to incline away from the gingival margin.

Fig. 4.10 Rotating Springs, clockwise (left) and counter-clockwise (right).

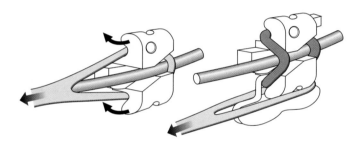

Fig. 4.9 Whenever retracting a single tooth, the risk of distal rotation is avoided by applying a light elastic force to a Power Pin instead of directly to the bracket (see text).

retraction (see Case 7). Using an elastomeric to a Power Pin, instead of directly to the bracket, reduces the risk of rotation, since the bracket is secured by its own elastomeric module, instead of by the end link of elastomeric chain, which will inevitably be stretched open by the traction (Fig. 4.9).

Rotating spring

The Rotating Spring™ is seldom required for correcting initial rotations. If this sounds a contradiction in terms, it is because rotations of anterior teeth are dealt with by full bracket engagement with light nickel-titanium wires, at the outset of treatment. (Premolar rotations are sometimes corrected with traction elastomerics, if bonded later in treatment.) However, the Rotating Spring can prove very useful for recapturing a rotation that has recurred in treatment, particularly if the patient is in a heavy archwire. The commonest instance will be if a ligature or a bracket has detached from a previously

rotated tooth. It is then convenient to be able to realign the rotation with the flexibility of an auxiliary spring, rather than having to delay treatment by stepping down to a lighter archwire.

Like the Side-Winder, the Rotating Spring comes in clockwise and counter-clockwise versions (Fig. 4.10), and is made in .014 inch high tensile stainless steel. Selection is simply a matter of viewing the tooth from the occlusal and determining in which direction derotation is required.

Although many operators use elastic ligatures in the normal way, there is a risk that ligature failure or stretch may allow the spring arm to displace the crown lingually. The former is rare, but the stretch of an elastic ligature should be guarded against by keeping activation of the spring light. The difference between wire or elastic ligatures is that a wire tie will limit the action to a perfect alignment, while an elastic ligature will allow some overrotation. Either way, the ligature should be placed first, before inserting the spring. It should also go without saying that adjacent space must be available into which the crown can align, since a light auxiliary spring cannot be expected to 'prise open' additional space in the presence of a solid archwire.

Strictly, a wire tie should only secure the archwire on the side of the bracket which is contacting the archwire (Fig. 4.11A); otherwise, if conventionally tied, the ligature will slacken as the instanding edge of the bracket advances to meet the archwire. Care should be taken to avoid running the ligature across the propeller slot, which will impede a complete correction.

To avoid occlusal interference, Rotating Springs should always be inserted gingivally, passed up the vertical slot with a light wire plier (Fig. 4.11B). Holding the spring arm directly to the labial, at 90 degrees to the tooth surface (less if used in

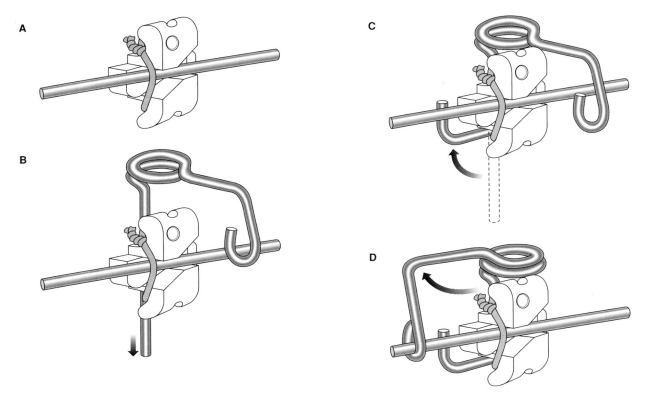

Fig. 4.11 Placement and activation of Rotating Spring. (A) The bracket is wire ligatured, crossing the archwire only at the side in contact. (B) A counter-clockwise spring is inserted from the gingival. (C) Pointing the arm of the spring directly away from the tooth (at 90 degrees to the tooth surface), bend the protruding leg gingivally in two right-angled bends (see text). (D) Hooking the arm around the archwire will now 'wind up' the spring and activate a counter-clockwise rotation (as seen from the occlusal). Squeeze the hook closed to prevent detachment.

conjunction with an elastic ligature), the long leg can be bent along the labial face of the tooth, to the same side as the hook will be engaged, the surplus end then tucking gingivally under the archwire (Fig. 4.11C). This contact of the leg against the crown ensures that when the spring arm is hooked over the archwire, the coils will be wound up to activate the spring. Finally, the hook should be squeezed closed around the archwire, using a Howe plier (Fig. 4.11D). Obviously, Rotating Springs are not intended for tackling severe rotations, when archwire engagement is not possible.

Just as with Side-Winders, Rotating Springs should only be used in conjunction with stainless steel archwires; anything less will be prone to labial deflection due to the action of the spring arm.

REFERENCE

1. Kesling PC. Tip-Edge Guide and the Differential Straight Arch Technique, 4th edn. Two Swan Advertising; 2000.

Treatment stages

Treatment stages

Differential tooth movement, as previously defined, involves repositioning of the crowns of the teeth first, followed by root uprighting to the new crown positions. However, there is a prescribed overall sequence of tooth movements, in the correction of any malocclusion with Tip-Edge, that needs to be followed closely. It is basically very simple and goes as follows:

- **Stage 1** is all about the anterior segments, which should be aligned, and any incisor spacing closed. They should also be corrected both antero-posteriorly and vertically (eliminating overjets, reverse overjets, increased overbites or anterior open bites). The archwires most commonly used will be .016 inch high tensile stainless steel, the resilience and flexibility of which is ideal for overbite reduction. Nickel-titanium auxiliary 'under arches' are frequently employed in the initial treatment visit, to assist in the alignment of instanding or rotated teeth.
  This first stage will normally be completed in between 6 and 9 months of treatment in Class II cases, considerably less in Class I and Class III cases.

- **Stage 2** concerns closure of any residual extraction spaces and seldom exceeds 3 or 4 months, except perhaps in first molar extraction cases. In non-extraction cases, it will obviously be very brief. However, it is important that centrelines should be coincident and correct before all the spaces are closed, since centreline discrepancies will prevent the attainment of a correct Class I occlusion. Also, the first molars require to be derotated in readiness to receive the rectangular archwires of the third stage.
  .020 inch high tensile stainless archwires are normally preferred during this stage, since they offer easy free sliding through the molar tubes, yet have enough flexibility to correct molar rotation. However, the extra robustness of

.022 inch wires may occasionally be indicated, such as when expanding maxillary crossbites, or in the lower arch when protracting lower second molars across a first molar extraction space.

- **Stage 3** is the root uprighting phase, during which each tooth is torqued and tipped to its preadjusted values, by the action of Side-Winder springs working against rectangular .0215 × .028 inch stainless archwires. Depending on the severity of the case, this may take up to 9 months to achieve. However, as pointed out previously, what was once a most complicated stage with the Begg appliance, has become virtually maintenance free with the new technology of Tip-Edge.

Buccal segment crossbites may be treated as a prior procedure, although this is seldom necessary, except perhaps in cases of severe transverse skeletal discrepancy. While the scope for crossbite correction in Stage I is limited by the light archwires used, it increases during the following stages with greater wire diameter, and particularly in the rectangular wire phase, when expansion can be supplemented by active torque control of the buccal segments.

It might be observed that the three stages outlined above broadly follow the Begg technique, although the method of achieving them may be considerably different, depending on the malocclusion type. Nevertheless, while Class II and Class III cases may treat towards the ideal result from opposite directions, with totally different vertical and anchorage considerations, the same stage sequence of objectives must always be observed. The overenthusiastic orthodontist who fails to do this by 'hitting everything at once', or improvising short cuts, will usually end up with increased treatment times and imperfect results.

CASE 1

A Class II 'Intermediate' malocclusion with mild crowding

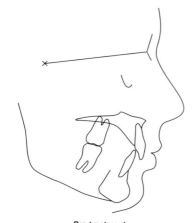

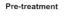

Pre-treatment

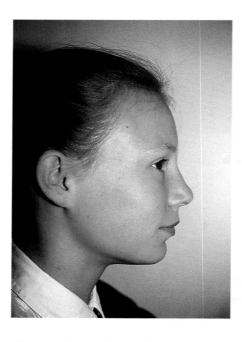

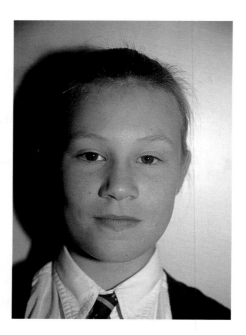

SKELETAL			TEETH		
SNA	°	79.0	Overjet	mm	5.0
SNB	°	74.5	Overbite	mm	5.0
ANB	°	4.5	UI/MxP	°	96.0
SN/MxP	°	7.5	LI/MnP	°	96.5
MxP/MnP	°	23.0	LI-APo	mm	-1.0
LAFH/TAFH	%	54.5			

1

At 13 years 8 months, a Class II intermediate incisor relationship with 4.5 mm of overjet, and a retroclined upper incisor segment. The lower incisors lie 2 mm behind the A–Po line. Skeletally there is a mild Class II base (ANB 4.5 degrees) with a reduced MM angle (24 degrees).

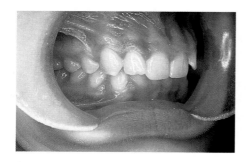

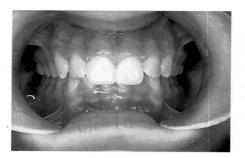

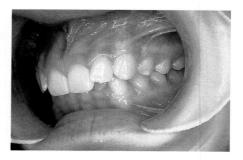

2

Both arches show mild crowding at the front. Because the mandibular angle is low, she will be suitable for light Class II intermaxillary elastics. The lower incisors are not proclined which, with a reasonable growth expectancy, invites a non-extraction approach. Since the overbite is increased and complete, anchorage bends to the first molars will maximize molar anchorage (see Chapter 7).

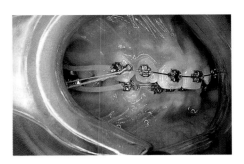
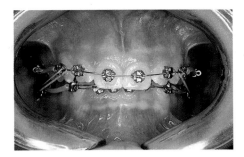
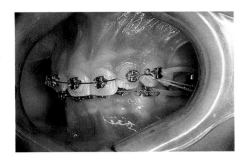

3

.016 inch high tensile stainless archwires are placed, with anchor bends mesial to all four first molars. A .016 inch multistrand underarch is employed to align the instanding lower lateral incisors. Because the overbite is deep, the premolars are left unbonded so as not to obstruct overbite reduction, and the round gingival molar tubes are used to maximize the effect of the anchor bends. To protect the premolar spaces, sleeves are placed between the canine brackets and the molar tubes. (Stops mesial to the molars would serve a similar function, but would detract from the resilience of the wire in reducing the overbite.)

Light (50 grams) Class II elastics are worn full time, changed daily.

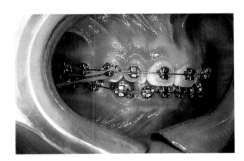
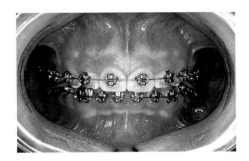
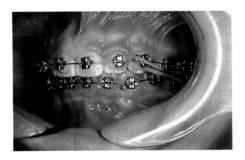

4

After 5 months, the overjet and overbite are reduced, with incisor contact above the lower incisor brackets. This signals the end of Stage I. The premolars are therefore bonded. The existing archwires are modified, removing the anchor bends in favour of vertical bite sweeps to maintain the reduced overbite. The archwires are now positioned in the rectangular buccal tubes, which will be used for the remainder of treatment.

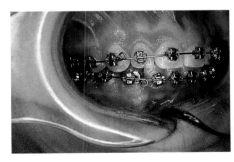
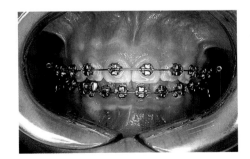
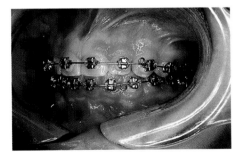

5

At the following visit, the premolars are aligned. .020 inch high tensile stainless archwires are fitted.

Stage II is brief in non-extraction cases, and is confined to derotation and levelling of the first molars, using offsets and toes, in readiness for the rectangular archwires at the next appointment.

Throughout the remainder of treatment, the interarch relationship will be maintained by the patient, wearing Class II elastics as much as necessary. Generally, in a co-operative patient, this amounts to no more than night times only.

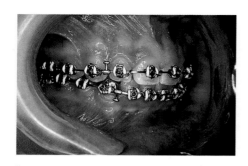
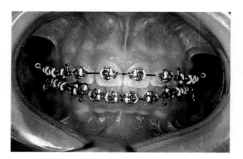
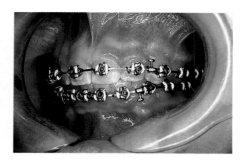

6
One month later, the .0215 × .028 inch rectangular archwires carry bite sweeps to maintain overbite reduction. Note how, unlike straight wire, the sweep is expressed at once, since it is not dependent on canine angulation. Pretorqued archwires are chosen, the pretorque cancelling out the proclination that would otherwise result from the sweeps, so preserving zero torque at the front.

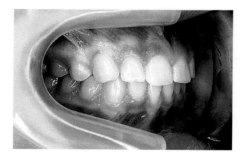
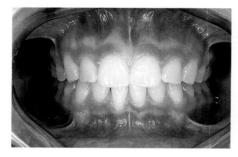
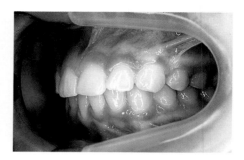

7
After 6 months in Stage III, the action of the Side-Winders is complete and the torque in base Rx-1 bracket prescription is fully expressed.

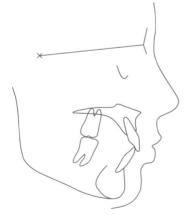

Post treatment

SKELETAL			TEETH		
SNA	°	78.0	Overjet	mm	3.0
SNB	°	75.0	Overbite	mm	1.5
ANB	°	3.0	UI/MxP	°	112.0
SN/MxP	°	7.0	LI/MnP	°	104.5
MxP/MnP	°	23.0	LI-APo	mm	2.5
LAFH/TAFH	%	55.5			

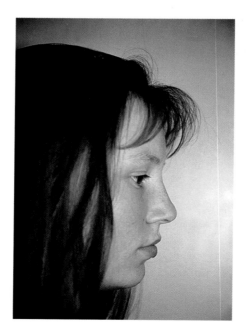
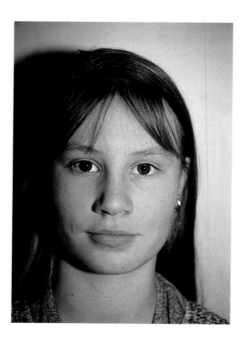

8
The lower incisors have advanced to 2.5 mm ahead of the A–Po line, with an improvement of facial profile.

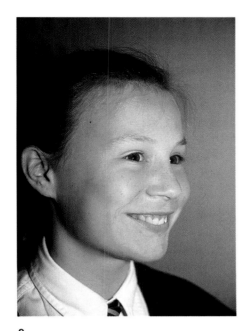

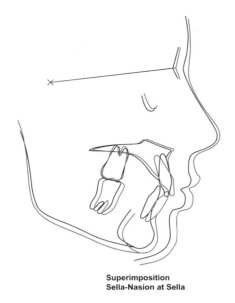

Superimposition
Sella-Nasion at Sella

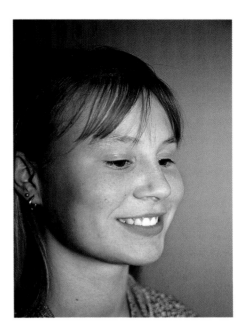

9
Growth has been small in extent, but has proved favourable. The upper central incisors have torqued 15 degrees and the gummy smile appears significantly reduced.

Treatment time = 1 year 3 months.
Routine adjustments = 10.
Archwires used = 6 (3 upper, 3 lower).
Retention = upper and lower Hawleys, nights only.

Bonding and setting up

Bonding and setting up

Since the Tip-Edge appliance is preadjusted, with a torque and tip prescription incorporated in each attachment, it follows that it should be set up just like any other straight-wire appliance. In this, the reader is referred to the work of Dr Lawrence Andrews, who was the originator of the preadjusted appliance and so defined the optimal bonding position for his crown related system.[1,2] This was designed around the best achievable reproducibility in bracket placement, based on easily visualized objectives, resulting in torque delivery that would prove consistent, irrespective of the size of the crown.

Bracket placement

A mid-crown position is therefore recommended for routine bonding. Each bracket should be aligned with its vertical axis parallel with the long axis of the tooth, and at the mid-point of the crown mesio-distally. The height of the bracket should be at the vertical mid-point of the fully erupted clinical crown (Fig. 6.1). All three dimensions are critical to an accurate end result, as with any preadjusted appliance, so that great care is required at the setting up visit.

Being a considerably smaller bracket than a Siamese twin type bracket has aesthetic advantages, but also makes the accurate placement of the Tip-Edge bracket rather more difficult, particularly on large clinical crowns. For this reason, Tip-Edge brackets are supplied with the option of coloured plastic jigs (Fig. 6.2). Not only do these provide ready 'sight lines' for the correct angulation of each bracket, but they also

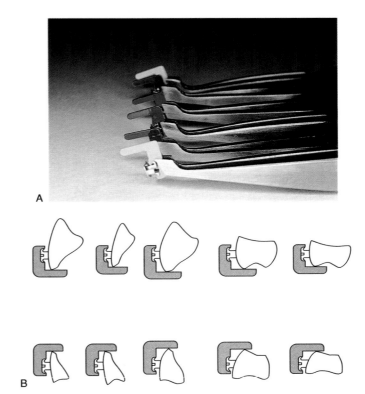

A

B

Fig. 6.2 Positioning jigs, as supplied, prescribe a fixed bonding height from the incisal edge, which is inappropriate to a preadjusted appliance.

make the brackets much easier to handle in conventional bonding tweezers.

Unfortunately, however, the jigs continue to be produced in 'L-shaped' form, which prescribes a fixed distance for each bracket from the incisal edge or tip. While this may have been appropriate for the Begg appliance, it is at variance with the requirements of a preadjusted appliance, in which the measurement of the mid-crown point to the incisal edge will vary according to the overall size of the crown. This problem can be solved simply by cutting off the horizontal sections of the jigs with ligature cutters, leaving only the straight vertical markers (Fig. 6.3). These can easily be aligned up the long axis of the tooth, while the mid-crown height can be gauged by eye (Fig. 6.4). On a normally shaped incisor, correct

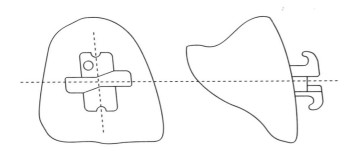

Fig. 6.1 Correct mid-crown bracket alignment (after Dr L.F. Andrews).

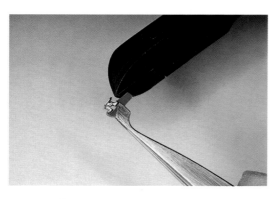

Fig. 6.3 Cutting off the occlusal rests allows freehand bonding to a mid-crown position.

angulation up the long axis will result in the incisal tie wing being parallel to the incisal edge of the crown.

The rationale behind a mid-crown bonding position is that the middle point of the crown is generally the point of greatest convexity on the curvature of the labial surface. It therefore follows that placing a pretorqued bracket further gingivally will decrease the torque prescription, while placing it too incisally will increase the torque. Reliance on L-shaped jigs, as supplied, frequently results in the latter. In addition, clinical experience shows that a true mid-crown position, as opposed to a more incisal bonding position, significantly reduces occlusal interference and hence cuts down on the number of accidental debonds, particularly on lower canines and premolars.

Overall, there are three major reasons why a bonding position further incisally is contraindicated:

1. The prescribed torque value in the bracket base is effectively altered, as described above.

2. For any given overjet reduction, the amount of retroclination produced during the initial tipping stage will be increased by siting the brackets towards the incisal tip. In turn, this will require an increase in the amount of root uprighting during Stage III.

3. When the Side-Winder spring uprights the root, in both tip and torque planes, during the third stage, it is placed at greater mechanical disadvantage if the distance between the point of rotation and the root apex is increased. This results in loss of efficiency.

Premolar brackets

Whereas anterior Tip-Edge brackets are designed to allow distal crown tipping during translation in the first stage of treatment, premolars may require to tip either mesially or distally, according to the extraction pattern. For instance, in a first molar extraction case, an upper second premolar will require to tip distally. However, if first premolars have been extracted, the same second premolar will need to tip mesially into the extraction space. Such situations are readily predictable, but might call for an unwieldy inventory of premolar bonds, in order to satisfy every possibility. The manufacturers have therefore simplified bond selection by using identical torque and tip values in upper first and second premolars, and similarly in the lower arch. In selecting the brackets, therefore, it is irrelevant whether it is a first or second premolar, left or right sided. All that the orthodontist needs to consider is whether the premolar is an upper or lower, and whether it will tip clockwise or counter-clockwise.

The notation on the bracket faces provides a simple check. Upper premolar brackets are identified by circular markings on the gingival tie wing, lowers by triangular markings, in the usual way. The occlusal tie wing carries an arrow (Fig. 6.5).

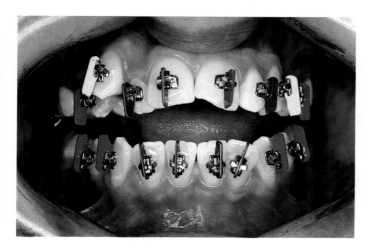

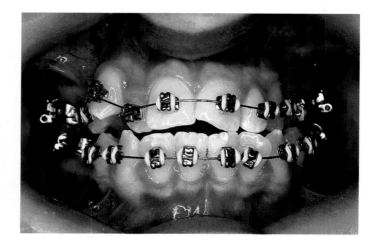

Fig. 6.4 Direct bonding with modified jigs.

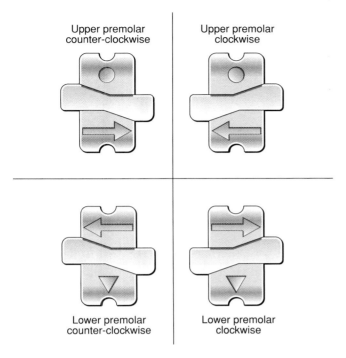

Fig. 6.5 Premolar brackets are selected according to the direction of mesio-distal tipping.

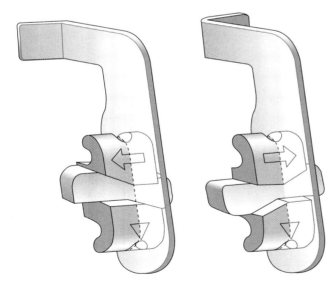

Fig. 6.6 The inclined tip of the 'Irish jig' on premolar brackets readily identifies the direction of tip, even when the arrow is obscured.

This indicates the direction of rotation. However, it has been found that when brackets are fitted with bonding jigs, these obscure the arrow, making it difficult to read the direction of rotation. For this reason, premolar jigs are modified by the addition of a 90 degree angle at the tip of the jig, which indicates the direction of rotation (Fig. 6.6). Because this problem was originally flagged up from Queen's University,

Belfast, it was perhaps inevitable that the modification would become known as the 'Irish jig'.

The various possible extraction patterns are illustrated (Fig. 6.7), from which it will be seen that the arrows invariably point towards the extraction site or, in a non-extraction case, towards the distal. In fact, as a rule of thumb, all the arrows point distally, with the exception of second premolars in first premolar extraction cases, as already mentioned.

In deep bite cases, as will be seen in the next chapter, premolar bonding is deferred until the end of Stage I.

Molar bands

With Tip-Edge, the use of bonded first molar tubes is contraindicated. This is because the withdrawal of the

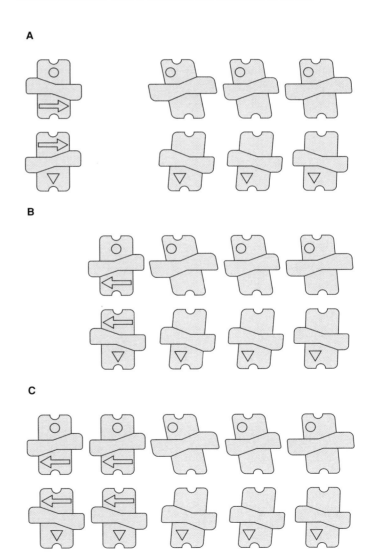

Fig. 6.7 Correct selection of premolar brackets for different extraction configurations: A = first premolar extractions, B = second premolar extractions, C = first molar extractions or non-extraction.

rectangular archwires at the end of Stage III is likely to cause bond failure. The extra security of molar bands is therefore recommended.

The rectangular buccal tubes should be aligned to the brackets, at mid-crown height, just as with a straight-wire appliance. The round tube will therefore sit towards the gingival margin. In the mandibular arch, the tubes should be parallel to the occlusal cusps; in the maxillary arch, however, seating the band fractionally higher toward the distal may be helpful in obtaining final seating of the disto-buccal cusp. It should be noted that round tubes can be omitted altogether in Class III malocclusions and cases with reduced overbites.

Second molars are not banded at the outset, except of course in first molar extraction cases, when they should be banded as just described for the first molars. Second molars are unnecessary to reinforce bite opening, contrary to straight-wire practice, and their inclusion in the early stages, particularly in extraction cases, merely adds friction. However, final alignment of second molars during the finishing phase is frequently necessary. If so, generally towards the conclusion of Stage III, conventional .022 × .028 inch rectangular tubes are used, either prewelded or bonded. Second molar tubes are available, although not specifically for Tip-Edge, with minus 14 degrees of torque and 10 degrees of distal offset (maxillary) and minus 10 degrees of torque and zero offset (mandibular).

REFERENCES

1. Andrews LF. Straight-Wire—the concept and the appliance. Wells Co, LA; 1989.

2. Andrews LF. The straight-wire appliance—explained and compared. Journal of Clinical Orthodontics 1974; 10: 174–195.

Stage I

Stage I

Objectives

1. **Alignment of upper and lower anterior segments.**
2. **Closure of anterior spaces.**
3. **Correction of increased overjet or reverse overjet.**
4. **Correction of increased overbite or anterior open bite.**
5. **Work toward buccal segment crossbite correction.**

The aims of the first stage are simply directed at correcting the anterior teeth, with the exception of centrelines, which do not require consideration until Stage II. However, the method of carrying out Stage I may vary considerably depending on the type of malocclusion, the skeletal pattern, age of patient and the degree of available space.

Anchorage mode

Since the Tip-Edge appliance has the capability of combining the treatment advantages of both Begg and straight-wire concepts, it has the flexibility to proceed in either mode, while exploiting the advantages of differential tooth movement. Anchorage may therefore be derived from a number of possible sources.

The principles of variable anchorage with Class II traction were first demonstrated by Dr Begg, and an evolved version of this works well with Tip-Edge in the treatment of most Class II malocclusions, particularly with increased overbite, and is dramatically effective in difficult deep bite cases. The reason for using Class II intermaxillary elastics in preference to headgear, wherever suitable, is ease of wear for the patient, leading to better compliance. Also, it is appropriate to say here that the side effects commonly attributed to Class II intermaxillary traction, such as clockwise rotation of the occlusal plane, opening of the mandibular angle and elongation of the upper incisors, while no doubt true with conventional fixed appliances, can be avoided with the use of such light forces as Tip-Edge allows in correctly selected cases.

Class I and Class III cases, without deep overbites, will frequently be treated by purely horizontal mechanics, as can be seen in Cases 7 and 8. Moreover, the high mandibular angle Class II facial type, as shown in Case 9, requires particular caution, avoiding any potentially extrusive

mechanics, such as Class II traction, which might risk the deleterious side effects mentioned above. In such situations, intrusive forces, as can be derived from headgear, can be used to advantage, to which Tip-Edge, being a light anchorage technique, is highly responsive. However, whichever way the case is approached, the objectives of the first stage always stay the same.

Because the maximum difficulty malocclusion, with increased overbite, uses the method least familiar to most orthodontists, this will be described here. It is effective in the treatment of the majority of Class II division 1 and division 2 cases.

The Class II case

A clinical case at the outset of treatment (Fig. 7.1) illustrates a Class II malocclusion with upper and lower anterior crowding and an increased overbite. Four first premolars have been extracted to gain the necessary space for overjet reduction and alignment. The mechanical principles in Stage I are therefore designed to align both anterior segments, concurrent with correction of overjet and overbite. To achieve this, .016 inch high tensile stainless main archwires are used, to control the molars and overall arch width, also to begin overbite reduction. Simultaneously, upper and lower sectional nickel-titanium 'underarches' provide the additional local flexibility for the alignment of the instanding incisors, in the initial treatment visits.

Vertical control of the incisor segments is by means of anchorage or 'tip-back' bends, placed 2 mm mesial to the upper and lower first molar round tubes. These will induce intrusion to both upper and lower labial segments as well as mesial root movement to the molars, so preventing loss of anchorage. It will be noted that the premolars are omitted from the appliance during overbite reduction. This is because the intrusive effect of the anchor bends mesial to the molars needs to be passed directly to the anterior teeth, without any vertical interference from the premolars in mid segment.

Overjet reduction proceeds concurrently, by means of light (50 grams) Class II elastics, worn full time, from the 'cuspid circle' hooks mesial to both upper canines, to the archwire ends distal to the lower first molar tubes.

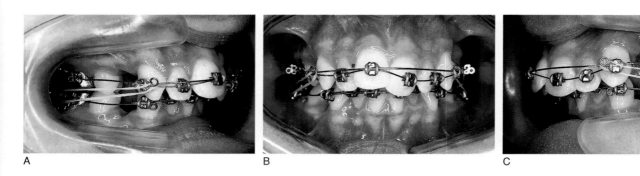

A   B   C

Fig. 7.1 Start of Stage I. In this severely misaligned upper arch, engagement to the main archwire is only possible with three anterior teeth, and the rotated upper right canine has a wire ligature safety tie through the vertical slot to prevent accidental disengagement. Beneath the .016 inch main archwires, the nickel-titanium underarches are .014 inch (upper) and .012 inch (lower).

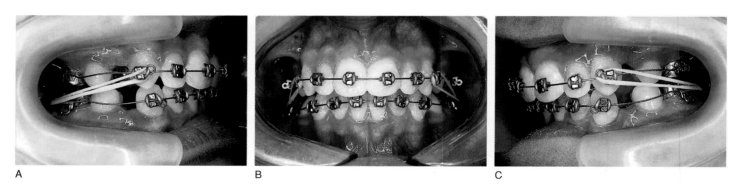

A   B   C

Fig. 7.2 Three months later, the underarches have been discarded. Because the labial segments are now in alignment, the canine brackets are ligated to the cuspid circles to prevent anterior spacing and archwire swing. Overjet and overbite reduction is ongoing.

It is seldom appreciated just how little force is required to move teeth, if the brackets allow them to tip. This answers the frequently raised question why the canines are not retracted first, in extraction cases. There is seldom need for this, since the canines are free to tip distally into the space available, and can slide along the archwire, without bracket binding, to permit decrowding of the incisors. This they do readily, in response to the instanding lateral incisors seeking space for themselves in the line of the arch. In the upper arch, control of the overjet is taken care of by the intermaxillary elastics, but even in the lower anterior segment, little transient proclination will result from rapid initial alignment. This is in marked contrast to conventional bracket systems, in which simultaneous bracket engagement on all crowded incisors will provoke proclination of the anterior segment, which may prove difficult to retrieve. The culprit is the canine which, if bodily controlled by an edgewise type bracket, effectively acts as an 'anchorage unit'.

After one or sometimes two treatment visits, the incisors will be aligned and the overjet and overbite partially reduced (Fig. 7.2). The nickel-titanium underarches have served their purpose and can be removed. It may be necessary to roll the cuspid circles distally along the archwire to regain their

position at the mesial of the canine brackets, which will have migrated distally to accommodate the instanding incisors. This is easily accomplished using the round beak of a loop-forming plier within the circle, as shown in Figure 7.3. Similarly the upper anchor bends will require periodic repositioning to the mesial, to prevent them disappearing into the molar tubes, as the archwire moves distally during overjet reduction.

Once the anterior segments are aligned, the canine brackets in each arch should be ligated around the cuspid circles on the archwire, in the manner shown in the next chapter, since further distal canine migration will not be required. There are two reasons why these ligatures need to be maintained during the remainder of Stage I:

1. They keep the six anterior units together as a block, not allowing space to enter the segment, as easily happens when teeth are allowed to tip.
2. They prevent the archwire from slipping from side to side.

Stage I is complete when the overbite and overjet have been reduced, with enamel to enamel contact achieved above the lower brackets (Fig. 7.4). This is the time to bond and align the premolars prior to Stage II.

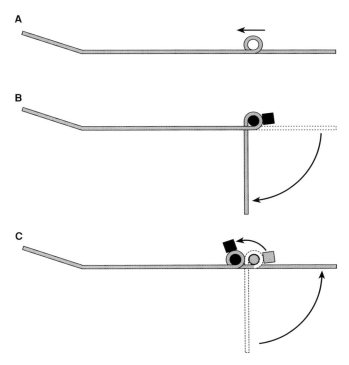

Fig. 7.3 Repositioning cuspid circle. To 'roll' circle distally (A), will require counter-clockwise rotation. First, unravel the anterior section the desired amount using a light wire plier (B), before winding up the posterior section to restore the horizontal (C). (Doing it in this sequence involves only a single section of wire within the plier throughout.)

Anchorage control

The above method illustrates the principle of variable anchorage, whereby the increased overjet and overbite are harmoniously resolved by a careful balance of forces (Fig. 7.5). Basically the six upper anterior teeth, being free to tip, comprise a light anchorage segment. By means of the Class II elastics, these are pitted against two lower first molars, which are maintained under bodily control by the mesial

apical influence of the anchorage bends in the archwire. These bends reciprocally encourage depression of the lower anteriors. The lower molars therefore 'dig their heels in' to resist the light mesial pull of the elastics, utilizing Dr Tweed's 'tent peg' principle for anchorage control, as described in Chapter 2. Similarly, the upper anchorage bends prevent mesial migration of the upper molars, by imparting mesial apical resistance. Care must be taken, however, to ensure that the elastic force is kept to a minimum, not exceeding 50 grams (2 ounces). Otherwise, the increased vertical component from too heavy an elastic can overwhelm the intrusive effect of the light maxillary archwire, and so elongate the upper anterior segment, as well as encouraging overeruption of the lower first molars.

Using this pattern of anchorage control, the assistance of second molars is unnecessary, either for overbite or overjet reduction. In fact, to include second molars in the appliance during the first stage is obstructive, as they create added friction during this and the space-closing stage.

However, consideration must be given to overall vertical consequences, and not simply to what we see happening in the mouth. Vertical forces imparted to the first molars by the anchorage bends need to be recognized. Clinical experience suggests that lower first molars extrude more readily than the uppers, no doubt due to the tip-back archwire bends and Class II elastics acting in combination, but also because of their more tapered root shape, compared with the triple divergent roots of maxillary molars. Obviously, therefore, it behoves the orthodontist to keep forces very light, which Tip-Edge readily permits. This requires a radical departure from conventional force thinking, familiar to the straight-wire and edgewise orthodontist.

Even assuming use of optimal light forces, whether or not the vertical reciprocals on first molars express as actual extrusion, will depend on the skeletal pattern and the attendant forces of occlusion generated by the 'muscular envelope'. In this, it is well recognized that the 'low mandibular angle' individual, with reduced lower face height,

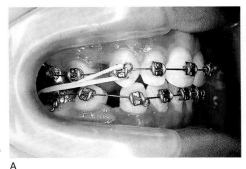
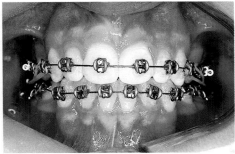
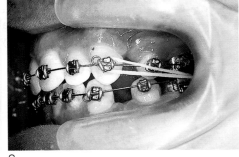

A   B   C

Fig. 7.4 Six months into treatment, the case shown in 7.1 and 7.2 has completed Stage I. The premolars are bonded in readiness for Stage II at the next visit.

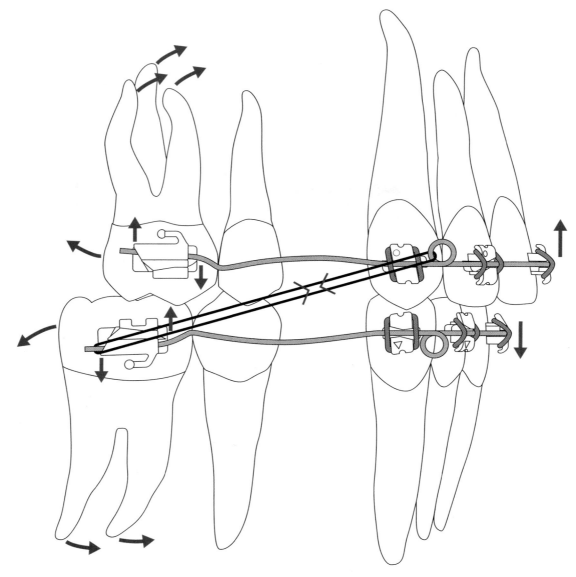

Fig. 7.5 Balance and distribution of forces during Stage I, when using Class II intermaxillary elastics and first molar anchorage bends.

has stronger musculature compared with the high angle facial type. It is the latter 'long face syndrome' case that is most vulnerable to extrusive forces to the posterior teeth, and for whom the treatment mechanics described above are therefore inappropriate.

Case 9 illustrates the use of intrusive mechanics in a high angle situation to control the vertical excess, and to correct 'gummy smile'. Examples of how to handle Stage I in various other malocclusion types are described in the relevant clinical cases.

A severe Class II division 1 malocclusion with crowding

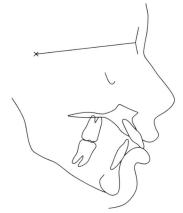

Pre- treatment

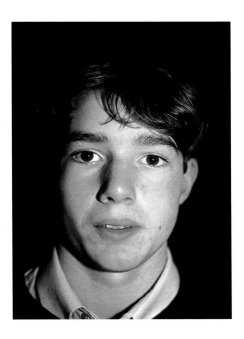

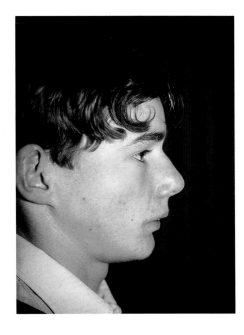

SKELETAL			TEETH		
SNA	°	81.5	Overjet	mm	12.0
SNB	°	76.0	Overbite	mm	4.0
ANB	°	5.5	UI/MxP	°	121.5
SN/MxP	°	5.0	LI/MnP	°	90.5
MxP/MnP	°	32.0	LI-APo	mm	-0.5
LAFH/TAFH	%	54.0			

1
At 14 years 9 months, a major overjet problem (12 mm) on a moderate Class II base (ANB = 5.5 degrees). Although the maxillary mandibular planes angle is slightly raised, the lower facial height is 54%. The patient is therefore potentially suitable for Class II intermaxillary traction. The lower incisors lie almost on the A-Po line.

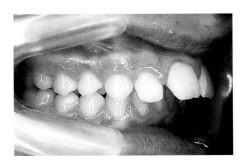

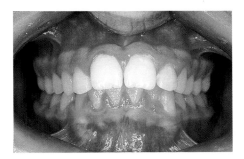

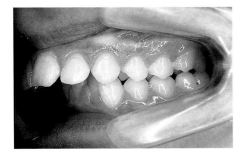

2
Whereas the upper arch is reasonably aligned, the lower incisors show some crowding, with an increased complete overbite. The extraction of upper first premolars is indicated to accommodate the reduction of this big overjet. However, with a light anchorage appliance, lower second premolar extractions are expected to give sufficient space for anterior alignment and levelling of the occlusal plane, as well as anchorage support for the overjet reduction. (Use of anchor bends in the treatment of deep overbite will greatly enhance molar anchorage.)

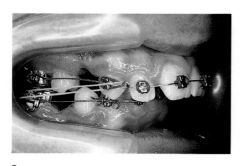 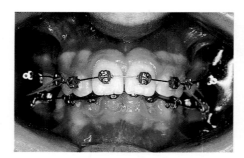 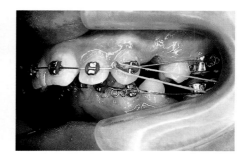

3

A typical Class II deep bite start, tackling the overjet, overbite and incisor alignment from the outset: .016 inch high tensile stainless archwires in round molar tubes with anchor bends mesial to all four molars. Fifty grams Class II elastics are worn full time. The premolars are omitted to facilitate overbite reduction. A .014 inch nickel-titanium underarch is engaging the lingually displaced lower lateral incisors and the lingually rotated lower canines are wire ligated for initial rotational control and security.

The cuspid circles are sited well mesial to the upper canine brackets so as not to prevent closure of the incisor spacing as the overjet reduces.

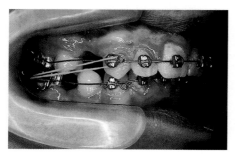 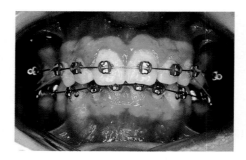 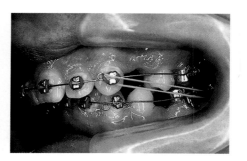

4

At the next appointment the overjet is down to 8 mm and the upper incisor spacing is closed. The lower laterals are aligned, so the underarch is discarded. The lower canine steel ties will be continued for a further visit to complete the derotation.

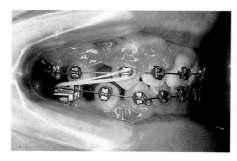 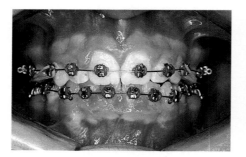 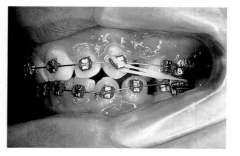

5

Four months into treatment, Stage I is complete: the overbite and overjet are corrected, with incisor contact above the lower anterior brackets.

The anchor bends are therefore discontinued in favour of bite sweeps, to retain overbite reduction. The premolars are bonded for alignment and levelling, so the rectangular molar tubes will now be used for the remainder of treatment.

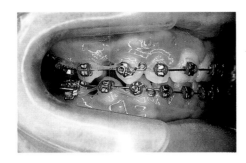 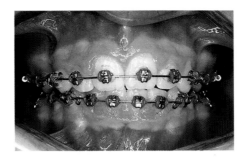 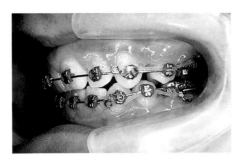

6

Stage II employs .020 inch high tensile stainless archwires with mild vertical bite sweeps to retain overbite reduction. There are appreciable extraction spaces to close in all quadrants. Tip-Edge offers the choice of doing this either by retraction or protraction. Clearly the anterior segments do not need taking back any further. Side-Winder 'brakes' are therefore placed on all four canines. With activation limited to about 45 degrees, these will exert gentle distal root movement to stabilize the anterior segments and thus ensure protraction of the posterior teeth into contact. The E-5 horizontal elastomeric links are routed though the premolar brackets to prevent detachment by 'fiddling'. Intermaxillary elastics will no longer need to be worn full time.

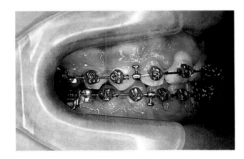 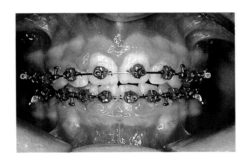 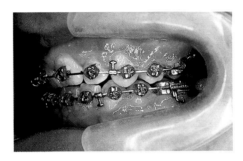

7

After 8 months, the latter half of treatment, once set up into Stage III, will be essentially maintenance free. .0215 × .028 inch pretorqued stainless archwires are selected, so as to preserve zero torque through the labial segments in the presence of continuing bite sweeps. Class II elastics only as necessary.

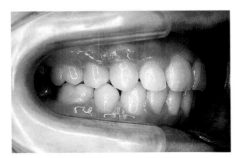 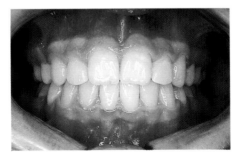 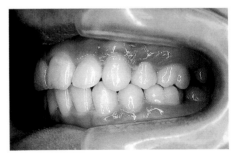

8

The Side-Winders have automatically delivered the Rx-1 torque and tip prescriptions to each tooth individually, against the zero torque base settings in the rectangular archwires.

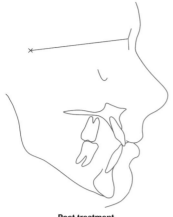

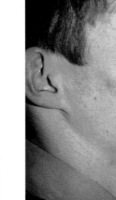

Post treatment

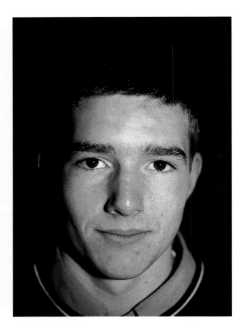

SKELETAL			TEETH		
SNA	°	77.0	Overjet	mm	2.0
SNB	°	76.5	Overbite	mm	0.5
ANB	°	0.5	UI/MxP	°	112.5
SN/MxP	°	5.5	LI/MnP	°	88.5
MxP/MnP	°	32.5	LI-APo	mm	3.0
LAFH/TAFH	%	55.0			

9
Easy lip control labial to the incisors will ensure stability of the reduced overjet.

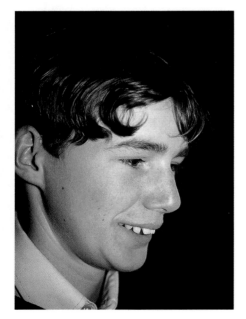

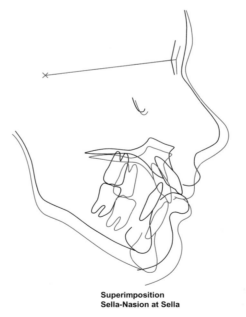

**Superimposition
Sella-Nasion at Sella**

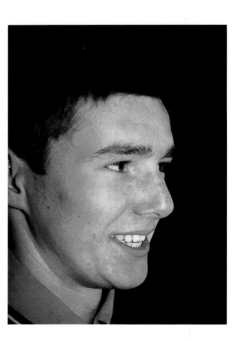

10
Favourable mandibular growth has carried the lower incisors downward and forward at similar angulation to a good aesthetic position 3 mm ahead of A–Po. Note good occlusal plane stability.

Treatment time = 1 year 5 months.
Routine adjustments = 11.
Archwires used = 6 (3 upper, 3 lower).
Retention = upper and lower Hawleys, nights only.

CASE 3

A severe Class II division 1 malocclusion with spacing

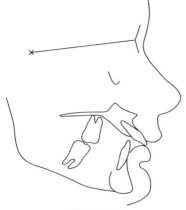
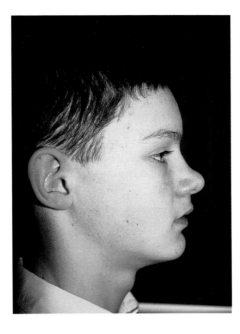
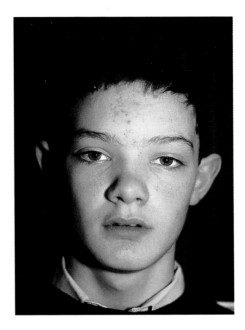

Pre-treatment

SKELETAL			TEETH		
SNA	°	81.5	Overjet	mm	11.5
SNB	°	79.5	Overbite	mm	0.5
ANB	°	2.0	UI/MxP	°	133.5
SN/MxP	°	6.0	LI/MnP	°	91.5
MxP/MnP	°	21.5	LI-APo	mm	-2.0
LAFH/TAFH	%	51.5			

1
At 13 years 4 months, a marked overjet of over 11 mm, but with considerable proclination of the upper incisors. The skeletal pattern is Class I (ANB = 2 degrees) and the low MM angle suggests suitability for Class II intermaxillary elastics. The lower incisors are 2 mm behind A–Po.

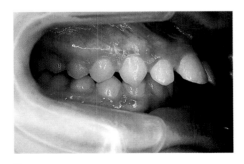
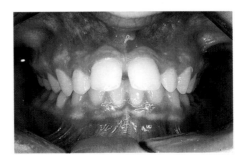
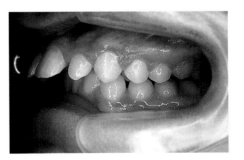

2
The upper incisors are considerably spaced, but the buccal segment occlusion will need appreciable correction, particularly on the left. As with Case 2, the presence of a deep overbite permits the use of anchor bends, thereby boosting molar anchorage. Premolar extractions are obviously not indicated and, despite the degree of overjet and interarch correction required, Tip-Edge offers a good expectancy that treatment goals can be achieved with light intermaxillary elastics, without recourse to headgear.

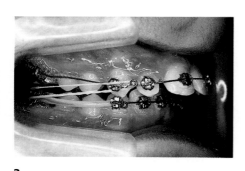
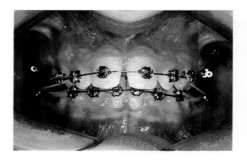
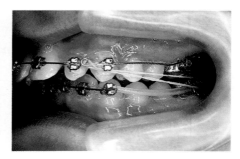

3

.016 inch high tensile stainless archwires with anchor bends mesial to the round molar tubes begin overbite reduction, while 50 grams Class II elastics reduce the overjet, largely at the expense of existing upper anterior spacing. Buccal sleeves safeguard the lower premolar spaces, whereas the upper premolars are presently spaced.

Note how the upper cuspid circles are positioned sufficiently mesial to the canine brackets to allow for anterior space closure. This could be achieved with a long intercanine elastomeric. However, in conjunction with Class II elastics, this is unnecessary, since the archwire will free slide distally through the canine brackets.

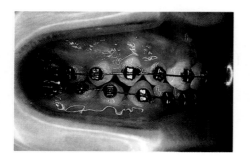
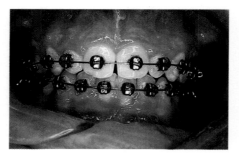
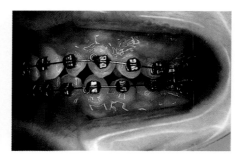

4

Four months later, the overjet and overbite are corrected. The premolars are picked up and aligned to the rectangular molar tubes. Anchor bends are replaced with bite sweeps. The buccal occlusion is not yet fully corrected, particularly on the left side. This is due partly to small upper lateral incisors, also the retroclination of the upper central incisors.

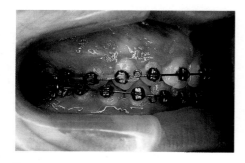
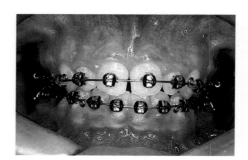
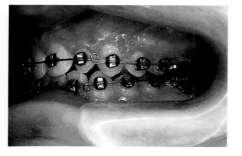

5

Stage II, in .020 inch stainless archwires, will consist mainly of correcting mesial molar rotations with offsets and toes, also levelling first molar distal crown tipping. However, a small amount of upper buccal segment space remains to be closed with E-Links® (TP Orthodontics Inc., La Porte, Indiana, USA) (E-6), concurrent with continuing Class II elastics.

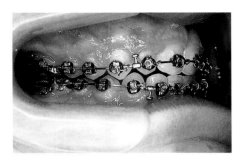
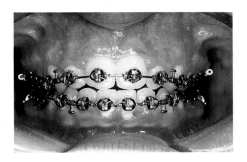
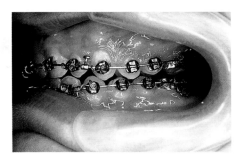

6

.0215 × .028 inch stainless rectangular archwires begin Stage III. Pretorqued archwires cancel out the proclination that would otherwise result from the bite sweeps, producing an overall zero torque base setting. Temporary bite 'propping' with Ketac cement to the upper first molars is needed to alleviate bite damage to the premolar brackets. Class II elastics will be necessary, on a part-time basis, particularly on the left side.

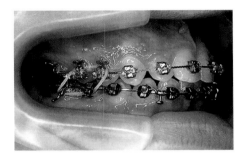
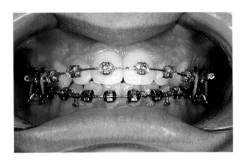
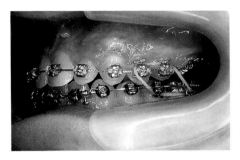

7

Torque and tip corrections are complete. In the final month of treatment, settling is achieved with an upper .019 × .025 multistrand archwire to the existing Stage III lower, wearing nightly 3/16 inch seating elastics in a 'Class II rhomboid' configuration, between gingivally inserted Power Pins and lower molar hooks.

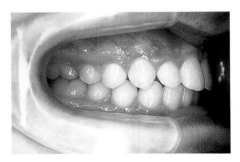
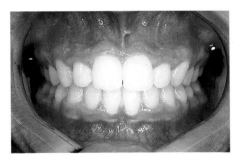
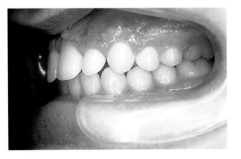

8

Treatment has been achieved without the use of headgear. Upper and lower second molars have been extracted to eliminate posterior crowding and allow the later accommodation of wisdom teeth.

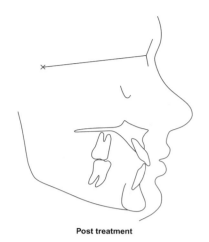

Post treatment

SKELETAL			TEETH		
SNA	°	81.0	Overjet	mm	3.0
SNB	°	80.5	Overbite	mm	1.0
ANB	°	0.0	UI/MxP	°	120.5
SN/MxP	°	6.0	LI/MnP	°	94.5
MxP/MnP	°	20.5	LI–APo	mm	1.0
LAFH/TAFH	%	52.0			

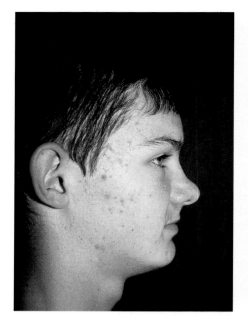

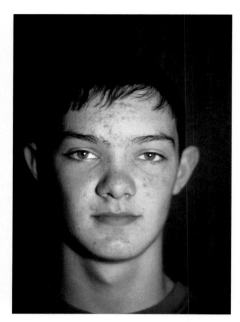

9
The profile has improved, with easy lip contact to retain the overjet reduction.

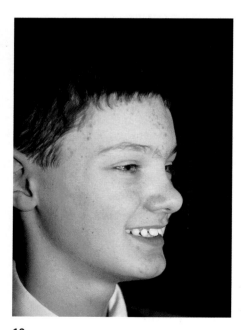

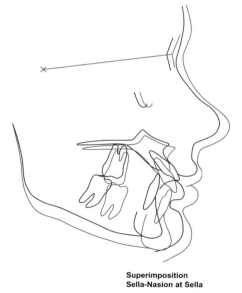

Superimposition
Sella-Nasion at Sella

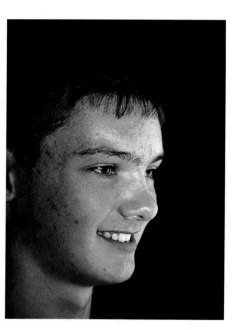

10
Mandibular growth has been good, with no opening of the mandibular angle. The lower incisors lie just ahead of the A–Po line.

Treatment time = 1 year 4 months.
Routine adjustments = 11.
Archwires used = 7 (4 upper, 3 lower).
Retention = upper and lower Hawleys, nights only.

Setting up Stage I

Setting up stage I

The following description shows how to set up a case along the lines illustrated in the previous chapter. The malocclusion features a marked increase in overjet, an increased overbite, plus severe upper and lower anterior crowding. The reader is invited to assume that the typodont does not have a significantly raised maxillary–mandibular planes angle or an increased lower facial height, and is therefore suitable for Class II intermaxillary elastic traction. Four first premolars are extracted (Fig. 8.1).

A question commonly asked is why such a case cannot be started more simply by means of nickel-titanium aligning archwires, before proceeding to stainless arches. The answer is that, while such wires do an excellent job aligning teeth, they are unable to control the vertical dimension and particularly the molars in the way that stainless steel can; neither can they support the use of intermaxillary elastics. The outcome would therefore be some loss of anchorage, by mesial molar migration, and a delay in implementing overbite and overjet reduction. Both are telling disadvantages in the more severe cases. Besides, with experience, the following method becomes easy to carry out and, once set up, is easy to adjust and maintain, without a change of archwires, over the 6 months or so necessary to obtain all first stage objectives.

The base archwire

.016 inch round high tensile wire is ideal for Stage I. This has the necessary resilience to withstand forces of occlusion, combined with the flexibility required to align mild tooth to tooth irregularities. It is particularly suitable for bite opening, offering a good range of action without excessive forces. The long established Special Plus grade Wilcock Australian wire continues to perform well, and more recently Bow-Flex® (TP Orthodontics Inc., La Porte, Indiana, USA) wire from TP Orthodontics (Fig. 8.2).

The 'horseshoe shaped' archform, as used in straight-wire techniques, is not appropriate for the early stages of Tip-Edge, since use of an anchorage bend requires a straight posterior leg. Combining a buccal archwire curvature with a vertical anchor bend will cause the wire to 'wriggle' and rotate within the buccal tube, which will invite a molar rotation. Even if an initial molar rotation is present, a straight leg is the rule. No

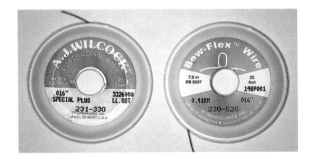

Fig. 8.2 High tensile stainless steel .016 inch wire should be used for the main archwires.

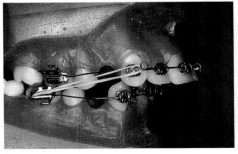

A

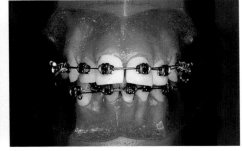

B

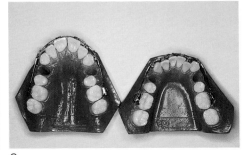

C

Fig. 8.1 Stage I—placement of initial archwires in a crowded case with increased overjet and overbite. Four first premolars have been extracted.

toe-in, in any shape or form, should ever be combined with an anchor bend.

The anterior curvature is interrupted by the 'cuspid circles', each of which should be placed mesial to its respective canine bracket. How close to the bracket will vary according to alignment and available space. If the labial segment is crowded, the canines will need to drift distally to accommodate instanding teeth, so that the circles may be immediately mesial to the canine brackets at the start of treatment. This will minimize the need for subsequent repositioning of the circles distally along the arch. Conversely, if the incisors are spaced, it makes better sense to site the circles further mesially, to allow for the mesial movement of the canines, relative to the archwire, as the anterior space is gathered up (see Case 3).

Once the anteriors are aligned and in contact, the correct position for the circles will be just mesial to the canine brackets. However they should not be more than 2 mm in front of the brackets, bearing in mind that in the aligned segment the circles will be ligated to the canines by elastomeric modules (as described later in this chapter) which, if too stretched, could provoke mesial canine rotations.

If bending an archwire up by hand, each circle should be formed so that the posterior section loops to the labial of the anterior segment and not vice versa. It should also be noted that the anterior archform curvature extends distal to the circles, across the face of the canines (Fig. 8.3).

When using Class II elastics and anchor bends, it is good practice to incorporate some overall expansion in the lower arch, as both components exert some elevating effect on the molar tube, which may cause lingual crown deflection. Five millimetres of expansion each side, measured across the molars, is generally adequate (Fig. 8.4), but this may be increased up to 10 mm in difficult deep bite cases. Even this does not amount to a strong expanding force in so light a

wire. Since the upper molars will not be carrying intermaxillary elastics, only a marginal degree of archwire expansion will be required here (Fig. 8.5), simply to counteract the effect of the anchor bend.

A considerable amount of clinical time can be saved by using preformed archwires, which are fabricated from .016 inch Bow-Flex wire (Fig. 8.6). These are size graded according to the distance in millimetres between the cuspid circles, which can be ascertained in the mouth with a flexible plastic ruler, between the mesial surfaces of both canine brackets (Fig. 8.7). As a check, the circles can be tried across the front of the mouth without inserting the posterior

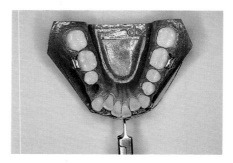

Fig. 8.4 Expansion of the lower archwire is advisable when using Class II elastics and anchor bends.

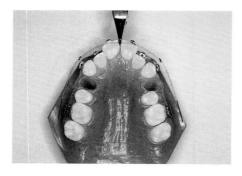

Fig. 8.5 If using anchor bends, a small amount of upper archwire expansion is needed.

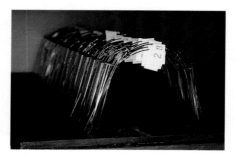

Fig. 8.6 Preformed .016 inch high tensile archwires save operator time.

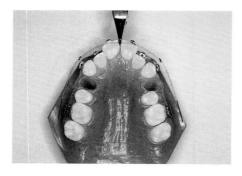

Fig. 8.3 Maxillary and mandibular archforms. Note the expansion of the lower.

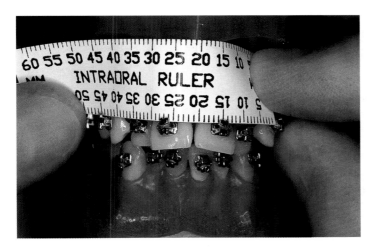

Fig. 8.7 The distance between the canine brackets determines the size of preformed archwire. Remember to compensate for any anterior spacing that may be present.

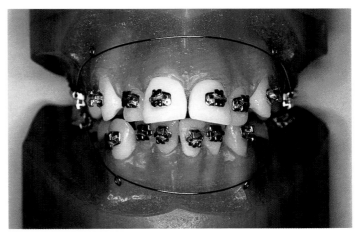

Fig. 8.8 Even this degree of active intrusion in a .016 inch archwire delivers less than 50 grams (2 ounces) intrusive force to each segment.

archwire legs, before removing the sticky identification label. Arch length and arch width can then be tailored accordingly.

Anchorage bends

Correct positioning of the anchor bends should be approximately 2 mm in front of the molar tubes in both arches. The most accurate way of finding this is to mark the archwire at the mesial of the buccal tubes, then remove the arch from the mouth and make each bend 2 mm mesial to the marks. Placing the anchor bends further forward than this will cause them to protrude occlusally and will slightly lessen the amount of overbite reduction imparted to the anterior segment.

The anchor bends not only boost the anchorage available from the first molars, but also exert vertical control. The degree of the bends is therefore significant to both. There is no hard and fast rule as to the angle of the tip backs, but each needs to be assessed by the amount of intrusive deflection that the archwire produces at the midline. In a case where there is little or no overbite reduction required, the bends can be minimal: just enough to prevent the lower molars tipping mesially. This may amount to only a couple of millimetres of active gingival deflection at the midline. However, in a low mandibular angle deep bite case, the anchor bends can be made to work harder and will correspondingly generate stronger molar anchorage. The maximum vertical deflection permitted in such cases can be to the depth of the labial sulcus (Fig. 8.8). Although this might appear somewhat extreme, the intrusive force distributed between the six anterior teeth amounts to only 2 ounces (or 50 grams) in the upper and rather less in the lower.

How many degrees of anchor bend will be required to achieve the desired amount of anterior arch deflection will also vary with the angulation of the molars. If the lower molars are tipped mesially, the amount of bend needed will

be reduced accordingly. In fact, at the outset of treatment, the mesial crown angulations of tipped lower first molars will sometimes provide sufficient anterior vertical deflection in themselves, without the addition of anchor bends at all.

Anchor bends should invariably be used in the round molar tubes, with the premolars omitted from the appliance.

The auxiliary arch

The round nickel-titanium underarch, usually of .014 inch diameter, has the task of aligning instanding anterior teeth,

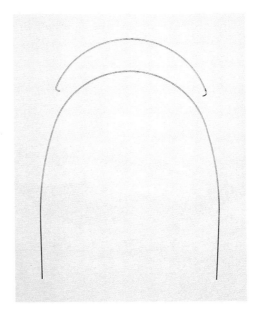

Fig. 8.9 The .014 inch nickel-titanium underarch should be cut from the anterior curvature of a preformed archwire.

and can usually be discarded at the first or second adjustment visit. It is best to use a curved section of wire cut from a preformed archwire (Fig. 8.9), rather than a straight section which might rotate about its long axis. This sectional auxiliary should extend 3 mm distal to the canine brackets. This facilitates use of the ligature gun (described later under Straight Shooter® (TP Orthodontics Inc., La Porte, Indiana, USA)) and ensures that the free end will not escape and flick out from within its elastomeric module. For patient comfort, the distal ends of the sectional should be turned 90 degrees to the lingual.

Fitting the arches

The auxiliary underarch goes in first, ligated to the instanding or rotated teeth (Fig. 8.10). With this in place, the tail of the main arch can be offered to the entrance of the round molar tube on one side (Fig. 8.11). This leaves a straight section of main archwire mesial to the canine bracket with the cuspid circle well clear, for easy use of the ligature gun. It also makes it easy to manipulate the underarch into the bracket, deep to the main arch, which holds it captive. Full bracket engagement of the canine is essential to security, particularly in the lower arch, and if this is not possible (usually due to a disto-lingual rotation) it may be necessary to use a wire ligature to the canine for the initial visit.

Once one canine is ligated, the buccal segment of the archwire can be slid distally to its true position, whereupon the opposite canine can be secured by the same means. Finally, the remaining incisors are zapped with the ligature gun (Fig. 8.12).

Sometimes an incisor can be so severely displaced lingually that it cannot be bracketed correctly at the start visit, in which case a bonded loop can be used initially. This can be discarded at the next adjustment, when a proper bracket can

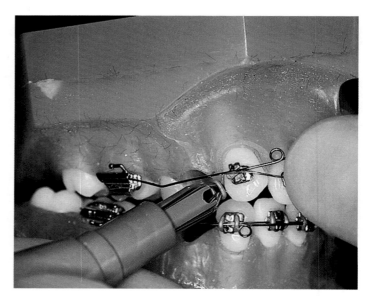

Fig. 8.11 Now insert the distal of the main arch into the entrance of the molar tube, on one side only. This facilitates ligation of the canine without interference from the cuspid circle, before sliding the archwire distally into place.

be placed. The nickel-titanium auxiliary arch can be loose tied if necessary, until full bracket engagement becomes possible. Alternatively, .020 inch elastic ligature thread can be tied around the main arch for preliminary alignment (Fig. 8.13). Although easier to insert, elastic thread tends to be unreliable and is less precise in the vertical dimension than an underarch.

Ligation of 'cuspid circles'

Mention was made in the previous chapter of subsequently ligating the canine brackets to the cuspid circles on the archwire. Obviously this is contraindicated while crowding exists in the anterior segment, as this would impede the distal canine migration described above, thereby preventing the alignment of the instanding incisors. However, once anterior alignment has been achieved, each canine bracket should be ligatured to its respective cuspid circle with an elastomeric, throughout the remainder of Stage I. As outlined in Chapter 6, this serves two purposes: the canines are prevented from further unwanted distal migration, so that the anterior segment will not become spaced; secondly, the archwire is stabilized laterally, and cannot swing from side to side. It follows that in a case with no irregularities in the anterior segment, ligation of the canines to the circles will be required from the very start of treatment.

There is, however, a right and a wrong way of applying the elastomeric modules to secure the canines. Simply engaging each tie wing and cuspid circle direct, following arch insertion, is incorrect, because the elastomeric will find its way beneath the archwire at the mesial of the canine (Fig. 8.14A).

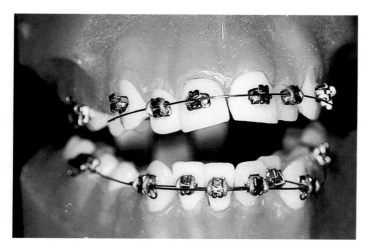

Fig. 8.10 Fitting the .014 inch upper underarch. Ligate the instanding incisors first.

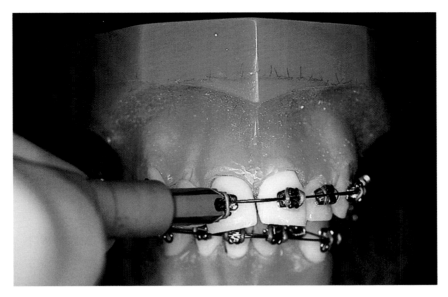

Fig. 8.12 Having done the same to the opposite canine, the remaining incisors are the last to be ligatured.

This may result in a mesial rotation, particularly if the elastomeric is under stretch. Figure 8.14B and C both eliminate this risk by providing labial archwire coverage at both mesial and distal.

Figure 8.14B is achieved by threading an elastomeric module on to the archwire from the back, before fitting the archwire in the mouth. The module should hang freely from within the cuspid circle (Fig. 8.15A). Then, following insertion of the archwire and ligation of the incisors (Fig. 8.15B), each module can be engaged around its respective cuspid bracket with haemostats (Fig. 8.15C). An

alternative method is the 'figure of 8' (Fig. 8.14C), sometimes known as the 'Swiss Twist'. This can be placed after archwire insertion. It is easiest to engage the cuspid circle first with haemostats, before twisting the elastomeric through 180 degrees and hooking it around the tie wings.

Anterior spacing

If the incisors are spaced at the beginning of treatment (unlike our typodont), they need to be approximated so that all six anterior teeth in the segment stand together as a block. An

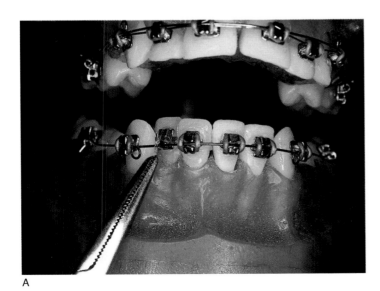

A

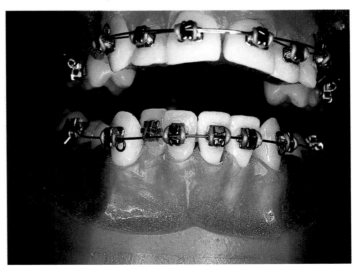

B

Fig. 8.13 (A) A big lingual displacement may initially need an elastic Zing String® (TP Orthodontics Inc., La Porte, Indiana, USA) tie through the vertical slot. (B) Once knotted, the tie can be rotated so that the knot hides beneath the bracket.

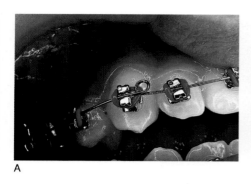
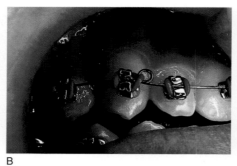
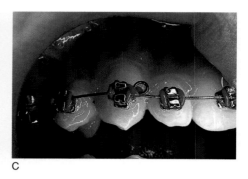

A

B

C

Fig. 8.14 (A) An incorrect cuspid tie. The elastic ligature lies beneath the archwire at the mesial. (B) A correct cuspid tie, with the elastic ligature labial to the archwire mesially, preventing mesial rotation. (C) Also correct, the figure of eight 'Swiss Twist'.

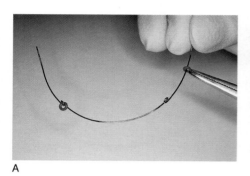
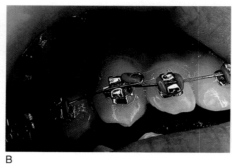
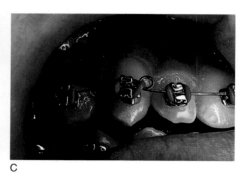

A

B

C

Fig. 8.15 (A) Before placement in the mouth, an elastic ligature can be slid along the archwire into the cuspid circle, from each distal end. (B) The cuspid tie lies loose within its circle while other brackets are ligated. (C) Finally, the cuspid tie is engaged around its bracket with haemostat 'mosquito' forceps.

elastomeric chain might be the anticipated method, but its force values are less easily controlled than elastomeric 'E-Links', which come in a variety of lengths. Generally a size E-9 is appropriate for closing upper anterior spacing. The end links engage the canine brackets, just as with chain, while the intervening span runs through the incisor brackets, deep to the archwire. The incisor brackets are retained with elastomeric modules in the usual way (Fig. 8.16). This is less conspicuous than chain, and easier to keep clean. In such a case, the cuspid circles must be sited well to the mesial of the canine brackets, otherwise these will act as stops on the archwire, preventing the canines from coming mesially.

If the amount of anterior spacing is relatively small, it may not require an intercanine E-link. The elastic ligatures from the canines to mesial cuspid circles will shrink minor spaces under only light stretch. Particularly if an overjet is present, as in Case 3, anterior space closure in the upper arch will happen anyway, due to the effect of the Class II elastics, without the help of an E-link.

The distal arch ends

Two millimetres of archwire should be left protruding distal to the lower molar tubes to accept the Class II elastics, and

should be bent about 30 degrees to the lingual for patient comfort. The upper arch ends can be cut immediately distal to the tubes. It is important not to cinch the ends gingivally, particularly in the lower arch. This is because any distal tipping of the molars in response to the anchor bends will drag the archwire distally, which will impart retroclination to the incisors (Fig. 8.17).

Intermaxillary elastics

These require to be worn full time from the upper cuspid circles to the distal ends of the lower archwire.

Why, it might be asked, should the distal arch ends be preferred to the more obvious molar hooks? There are two reasons: firstly, the vector of elastic force is more horizontal when used in this way, since use of the hook increases the undesirable vertical vector of elastic force by being both further forward and more gingivally placed (Fig. 8.18). (The difference becomes even greater in extraction cases, when spaces close and arch length shortens.) Secondly, overbite reduction is arguably more effective with a more distal application of elastic to the molar, which better resists distal crown tip and therefore encourages a fuller expression of the anchor bends to the anterior segment.

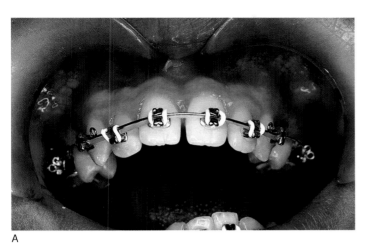
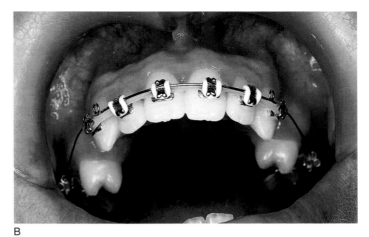

Fig. 8.16 (A) An E-9 intercanine elastomeric to close upper anterior spacing. (B) One month later.

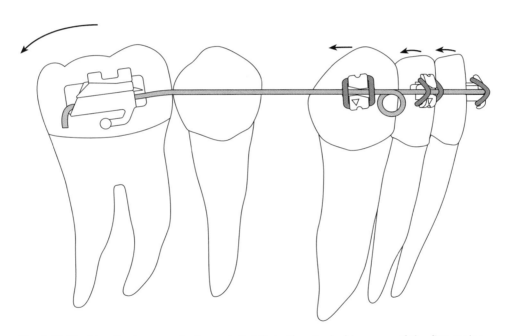

Fig. 8.17 Cinching the lower archwire ends tightly to the gingival is wrong. If the first molar tips distally due to the anchor bend, it will drag the lower labial segment lingually.

It is absolutely essential to keep the elastic force light at all times. 50 grams or 2 ounces each side may be as little as one sixth of that recommended by some straight-wire orthodontists, and is of course one major reason why Tip-Edge can escape the unwanted side effects of intermaxillary elastics, as explained previously. However, it needs to be stressed again that using forces in excess of 50 grams with Tip-Edge increases the risk of elongating the upper incisors, by overcoming the intrusive effect of the upper anchor bends, as well as provoking problems of lower molar control. The Tip-Edge orthodontist quickly learns the value of light forces, and will soon recognize that slow progress, if it occurs, is the result of poor compliance with the elastics, rather than inadequate forces.

Ligatures

Steel ligatures are only occasionally necessary in Tip-Edge, and then only at the start of treatment (or if using a derotating spring). An interim steel tie may initially be a safeguard against disengagement, where the archwire cannot be fully seated, or to obtain full bracket engagement of a nickel-titanium underarch on a rotated tooth. However, these should

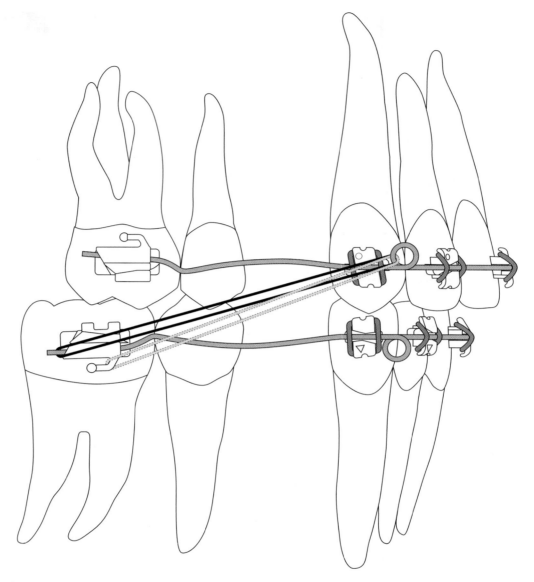

Fig. 8.18 There is a significant difference between the vertical force vector produced by Class II elastics worn to the distal arch end as opposed to the molar hook. The distal arch end is better.

be substituted for elastomeric ligatures as soon as possible, since the relative inflexibility of steel ligatures inhibits the free tipping of the brackets, and is therefore liable to increase anchorage in the wrong places.

'Straight Shooter'

This ingenious ligature gun is ideally suited to Tip-Edge, but can also be used with many edgewise type brackets. With experience, it convincingly upstages the traditional haemostat forceps for placing elastomeric modules, and greatly speeds adjustment visits throughout Tip-Edge treatment.

Made from autoclavable plastic (similar to that used on wingtips of supersonic aircraft) each elastomeric module is picked up from a flat surface or an adhesive Stickyring® (TP Orthodontics Inc., La Porte, Indiana, USA) (Fig. 8.19). The Straight Shooter should be placed over the bracket, at right angles to it, while progressively squeezing the trigger (Fig. 8.20). This separates the four claws to stretch the module around the outside of the tie wings (Fig. 8.21). At this point, the trigger is squeezed fully (Fig. 8.22), advancing the inner piston to expel the module from the claws, allowing it to contract securely around the tie wings (Fig. 8.23).

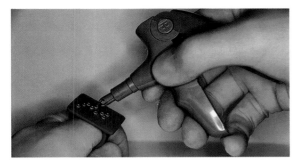

Fig. 8.19 The Straight Shooter picks up from a flat surface (or Stickyring).

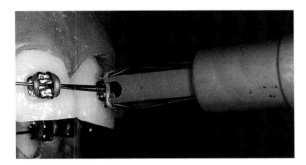

Fig. 8.20 The claws open as the trigger is squeezed.

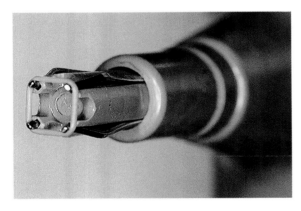

Fig. 8.21 The module is stretched around the tie wings.

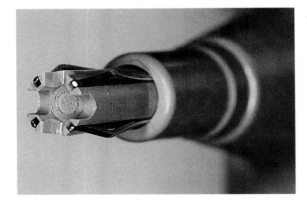

Fig. 8.22 The piston ejects the module.

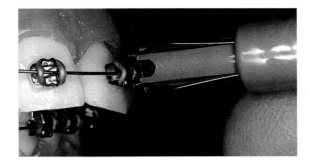

Fig. 8.23 . . . which contracts around the tie wings. Eureka!

Apart from speed in use, the ligature gun places less pressure on the tooth than when stretching a module around a bracket by hand. It is therefore more comfortable for the patient and needs less concentration from the operator. There is also less risk of an accidental 'gingivectomy' by slipping off the bracket! Initially, however, it requires familiarization. It takes a few weeks of regular use to become an expert 'marksman'.

Instructions for intermaxillary elastics

As orthodontists, we need to recognize that communication is of paramount importance in obtaining the co-operation of our patients. An appreciation by the patient of what is going on is essential to good compliance. Since intermaxillary elastics will be the 'power source' in the majority of Tip-Edge cases, a thorough explanation of their use is time well spent at the set-up visit. Otherwise, particularly as the elastic forces are so light as to be hardly perceived by the wearer, the patient may be tempted to regard them as an 'add-on' to treatment, rather than the primary motive force.

The author's policy is to explain that the archwires do the straightening and provide a guidance pathway for the front teeth to follow, but actual movement of the front teeth backwards is done entirely by the patient, by wearing the elastics full time. A simple explanation of tooth movement follows, emphasizing that even very light elastic messages will signal the teeth to begin moving after 24 hours or so, whereas leaving the elastics off for even an hour will halt the process entirely, requiring many additional hours of wear to restart it. While not strictly true physiologically, this does impress upon the patient the big difference in progress resulting from 100% as opposed to 90% wear. The fact is that a 90% wearer will all too easily drop to 80%, and so on.

The patient is given two packets of elastics, one to be used for routine replacement every night before bed time, the other to be carried with them wherever they go, for instant replacement in the event of loss or breakage, much as every car carries a spare wheel in case of a puncture. The elastics should only be removed for cleaning the teeth.

Every orthodontist will have his or her own way of reinforcing the message. An excellent protocol from a leading Tip-Edge practitioner (C.C. Twelftree, personal communication) goes as follows:

Patients are told to wear elastics all the time, even when eating. They may remove the elastics for cleaning only, but the elastics must be placed over a finger during this time. If elastics are placed on the basin or the end of a tooth brush they will occasionally be forgotten. I require elastics to be changed only when they break, to minimize force values, and this means that two or three elastics need to be kept with the patient at all times. These can conveniently be carried on a watch band or a safety pin. At the first appointment after appliance insertion, which is always 1 week later, the patient is intelligently quizzed regarding elastic wear to re-emphasize the instructions.

Stage I checks

Stage I checks

The routine adjustment interval throughout Stage I is 6 weeks. At each adjustment visit, the following checks will be necessary:

- **Measure the overjet.** The normal expectation for overjet reduction in extraction cases will be 3–4 mm per visit. Non-extraction cases and adults may be a little slower. *Failure of overjet reduction is almost invariably due to partial elastic wear, which can be further confirmed by distal crown tipping of the lower first molars, since the anchor bends will no longer be balanced by the mesial elastic forces. Occasionally, the archwire ends protruding distal to the upper first molars may impact against buccally displaced upper second molars. If so, they should be shortened.*

- **Observe the overbite.** The incisor overbite may take a visit or two to respond and the rate of overbite reduction varies according to the skeletal pattern and age of the patient. *If the overbite fails to reduce, the cause will be either poor elastic wear, as described above, or damage to the anchor bends. The latter can be checked by releasing the archwire from the anterior segment, while keeping it engaged in the molar tubes. The amount of vertical activity remaining in the wire at the front can then be observed.*

- **Molar widths.** These should be checked with dividers. *Lingual contraction of first molars suggests that the anchor bends are too strong, or that the archwire has been inadequately expanded. In the mandibular arch, it may also denote use of excessive elastic force. (In first molar extraction cases, lingual rolling of the banded second molars may require the patient to wear the Class II elastics to lingual hooks on the second molars by night, conventionally by day.)*

- **Check the cuspid circles.** Attention to these is generally only necessary during the initial treatment visits, when the incisors are being decrowded or anterior spacing closed. *If anterior space is refusing to close, the cuspid circles may be preventing the canines from being gathered into contact with the incisors, and will need rolling mesially. In severely crowded cases, the canine circles may require to be rolled distally to catch up with the canines, which will have migrated backwards to allow the accommodation of crowded incisors.*

- **Siting of anchor bends.** These should be maintained 2–3 mm in front of the molar tubes. Particularly during overjet reduction, the upper anchor bends are likely to need repositioning forwards, as the archwire slides distally through the molar tubes. *Allowing an anchor bend to enter a molar tube will cause binding.*

- **Distal arch ends.** For similar reasons, the arch ends distal to the molar tubes may lengthen and require trimming. Equally, it is important to make sure that each distal end is plainly visible and not too short. *If a distal arch end fails to protrude beyond the distal of the tube, it will generate friction within the tube and prevent free sliding.*

- **Distortion of the archwire.** This requires removal of the wire to assess accurately and rectify. The anchor bends should be reinstated to produce the correct degree of anterior intrusion. *A negligent patient should be cautioned to avoid hard substances, as repeated biting out of the tip-back bends will result in reduced anchorage resistance from the molars, as well as poor overbite reduction.*

- **Reassess the elastic tension.** As intermaxillary elastics take effect, the distance between the attachment points will inevitably reduce, resulting in a lesser degree of stretch. It will therefore be necessary to check the elastic forces on a strain gauge, and against clinical progress, replacing them with a smaller size if necessary, in order to maintain the ideal tension (50 grams or 2 ounces).

'Power Tipping'™

'Power Tipping'™

The danger of proclining lower incisors undesirably during overbite reduction, particularly where anterior crowding is present, must be recognized with any appliance. With Tip-Edge, as previously explained, projecting the lower front teeth labially during decrowding is less likely than with straight-wire type appliances, because the lower canines are not held bodily by the bracket, and are therefore free to tip distally along the arch into available space.

The situation becomes more threatening, however, in the case of overbite reduction in an already proclined lower incisor segment. Here, by the simple laws of physics, it will be understood that the intrusive force from an archwire within a labially placed bracket acts along an axis that will be considerably labial to the centre of rotation of a proclined incisor (Fig. 10.1). If further proclination is to be avoided, a lingual component of force must be introduced to counteract the proclination. How might this be done?

In a conventional edgewise derived bracket, lingual incisor crown torque might be induced by means of a torqued rectangular archwire, assuming that the anteriors are sufficiently aligned to permit full bracket engagement. However, Tip-Edge

brackets cannot achieve third order torque against rectangular wire while in transitional angles of tip. It would, of course, be easy enough to generate lingual crown movement by the simple expedient of adding intramandibular traction along the arch, but this would introduce a reciprocal mesial force to the lower first molars, thereby dragging molar anchorage.

A much better way is 'Power Tipping™', as illustrated in Case 4. Power Tipping is simply applied with virtually no loss of anchorage. It can be used to the existing Stage I archwire, and does not need to wait until incisor alignment is complete.

How does it work?

Power Tipping utilizes 'reverse Side-Winder springs' to induce distal crown torque to the lower canines, and hence distal retraction, which in turn uprights the lower anterior segment lingually (Fig. 10.2). It is essential to ligate the canine brackets to the cuspid circles during this process, assuming the anterior teeth are in alignment; otherwise the canines will retract along the arch without taking the lower incisors lingually, like a locomotive leaving its train behind. Obviously, use of Power

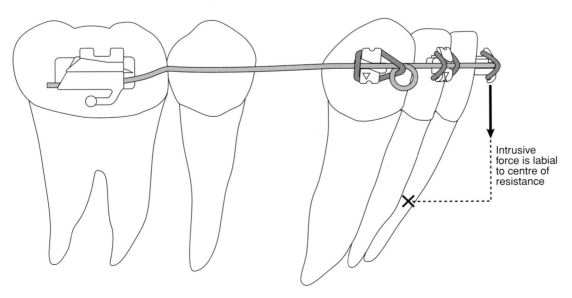

Intrusive force is labial to centre of resistance

Fig. 10.1 An archwire exerting an intrusive force on an already proclined incisor may cause unwanted further proclination.

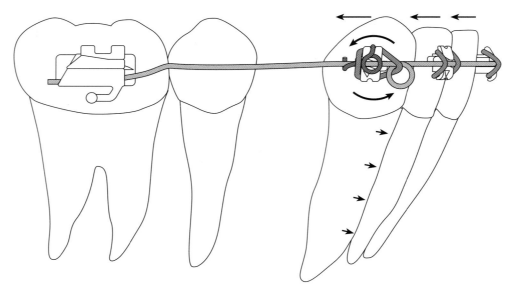

Fig. 10.2 Addition of Power Tipping to the lower canines induces lingual movement of the lower labial segment, by means of distal crown movement of the canines.

Tipping presupposes that there is available space in the arch to the distal, into which the canines can migrate. If not, mesial root movement of the canines will result, instead of the distal crown movement intended. Power Tipping can be applied at any time during Stage I, when it becomes apparent that unwanted proclination is developing during overbite reduction. It does not require modification of the archwire.

The clinical scenario illustrated (Fig. 10.3) shows Stage I in progress during the treatment of a 12 mm overjet with a complete overbite in which the lower incisors were initially proclined, and now threaten to procline further under the intrusive influence of the anchorage bends, coupled with the use of Class II elastics. Four premolars have been extracted and the Stage I assembly is as described in previous chapters, using .016 inch high tensile stainless archwires with anchor bends to the round buccal tubes. The premolars are omitted.

The addition of Power Tipping consists merely of inserting Side-Winder springs into the lower canine brackets. Since Power Tipping is designed to induce distal crown tip, rather than to correct it, the springs are fitted in the reverse direction to that in which they will be used later, in Stage III; in other words, the lower right canine will use a counter clockwise spring, and the left canine a clockwise version. Note that both canines are secured to the cuspid circles by elastomerics.

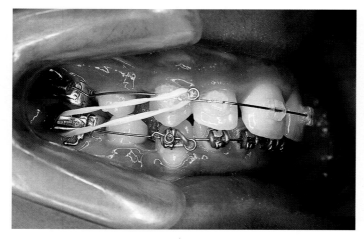

Fig. 10.3 Power Tipping applied to lower canines. Note the cuspid tie necessary to prevent each canine escaping distally without taking the incisors lingually.

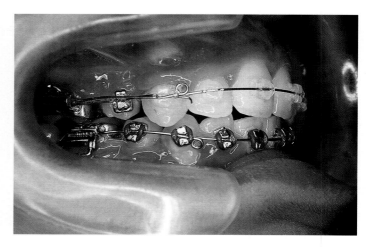

Fig. 10.4 Four months later, the lower incisors have been uprighted lingually.

Used in this way, the auxiliary springs may be regarded as little 'motors', gently propelling the crowns backwards by distal rotation which will, due to the canines being tied to the cuspid circles, cause the incisors to tip lingually as required. Full activation of the Side-Winders is not necessary to achieve this: about 45 degrees of activation is generally sufficient.

Four months later (Fig. 10.4), the lower anterior segment has inclined lingually, despite the full time Class II elastics, due solely to the influence of the reverse Side-Winders. The clinical response does not appear to vary significantly according to whether first or second premolars have been removed. The same method can be used in non-extraction cases, only so long as there is available space mesial to the molars.

The principle of moving crowns by the application of root forces is by no means unique to Tip-Edge. While straight-wire appliances cannot employ Power Tipping electively in the present context it is, for example, accepted practice to assist buccal segment expansion with active buccal crown torque. It might be reasoned that Power Tipping induces some unwanted mesial apical movement on the lower canines, which must later be reversed. No doubt this is so, but radiographic observation suggests that the degree of mesial root movement is very slight, compared with the amount of distal crown tipping obtained. Arguably the process is virtually 'anchorage free', particularly since no mesial forces are imparted to the first molars.

CASE 4

A Class II division 1 malocclusion with mild crowding and marked bimaxillary protrusion

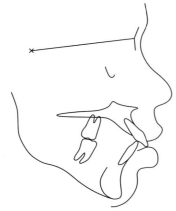

Pre-treatment

SKELETAL			TEETH		
SNA	°	80.0	Overjet	mm	8.0
SNB	°	77.5	Overbite	mm	3.0
ANB	°	2.5	UI/MxP	°	123.0
SN/MxP	°	2.0	LI/MnP	°	97.5
MxP/MnP	°	35.5	LI-APo	mm	8.0
LAFH/TAFH	%	56.0			

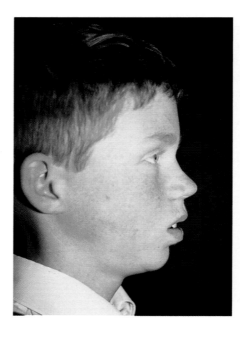
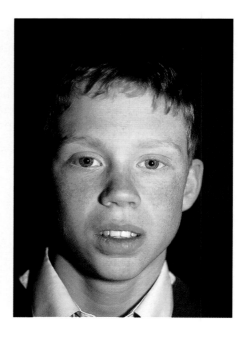

1

At 12 years 11 months, the overjet measures 8 mm and the lower incisors are proclined 8 mm beyond the A–Po line. Skeletally mild Class II, there is some increase in the MM angle (35 degrees) and lower face height (56%). However, this is not 'a long face syndrome', and will hopefully be suitable for Class II elastics, provided the lower anchor bends are kept light, to prevent molar extrusion.

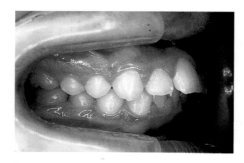
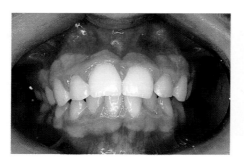
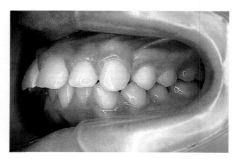

2

Upper arch alignment is reasonable but the lower incisors show mild crowding. Four first premolar extractions are indicated here, because the lower incisors are 8 mm in front of A–Po and the present 8 mm overjet will need reducing to a somewhat lingually corrected lower incisor position.

The expectation that such objectives can be met simply with Class II intermaxillary mechanics is a reflection of a low anchorage bracket system.

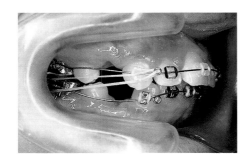
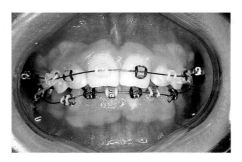
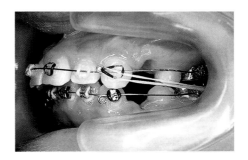

3

Stage I begins with .016 high tensile stainless archwires with light anchor bends to the round molar tubes. Because of the deep overbite, the premolars are left unbonded. Fifty grams Class II elastics will reduce the overjet. No underarch is required, but the elastomeric modules to the lower lateral incisors are under slight stretch. For this reason, the lower canine brackets are not ligated to the cuspid circles, so that the canines are free to ease distally, to make room for the laterals.

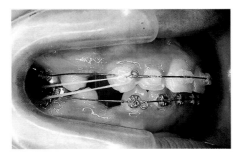
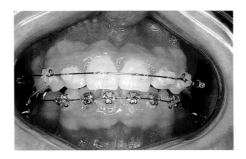
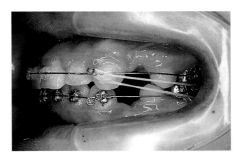

4

At the following adjustment, the overjet and overbite are reducing well and the lower incisors are aligned. However, there is a risk that the lower incisors may procline further as the overbite continues to reduce. This is because an intrusive force is being applied to a labial bracket system on an already proclined tooth, as described in Chapter 10.

Power Tipping is therefore applied to both lower canines by means of reverse Side-Winders, with activation reduced to approximately 45 degrees. The gentle mesial root moment will translate into a distal crown rotation along the arch. Note that each canine must be ligated to its cuspid circle, otherwise the canines will motor off distally, leaving the incisors behind.

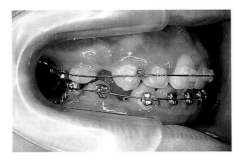
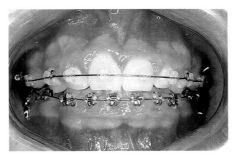
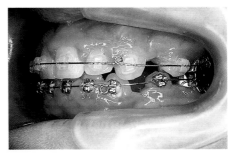

5

Five months into treatment, the overjet and overbite have reduced to the new lower incisor position. See how the lower incisors have retroclined over mandibular base, due to the Power Tipping. The Side-Winders are removed, and the premolars are aligned to the rectangular tubes with the existing archwires, bite sweeps replacing the anchor bends.

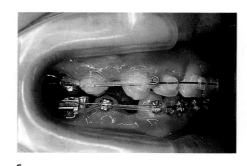
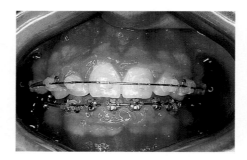
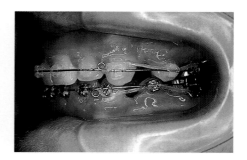

6

Next visit, Stage II .020 inch stainless archwires begin space closure with horizontal elastomerics in all quadrants (E-6). Because the lower incisors were so procumbent initially, this is a retractive Stage II with no brakes required (see Chapter 11).

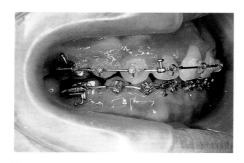
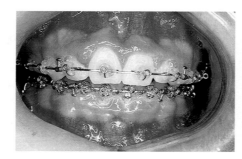
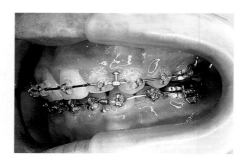

7

Repeated bite damage to the lower canine brackets has necessitated set downs in the .0215 × .028 inch archwires. Otherwise these are standard Stage III pretorqued archwires, maintaining an overall zero torque setting in the presence of the sweeps needed to retain the reduced overbite. Class II 'check' elastics will be worn at nights to promote molar occlusion (see Fig. 18.4).

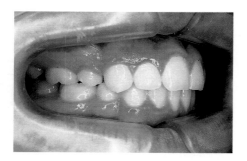
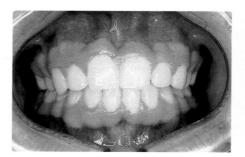
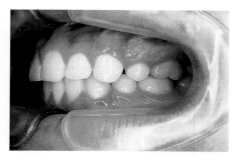

8

Treatment is complete after 7 months in Stage III.

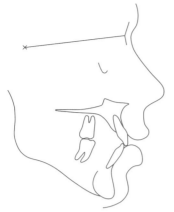
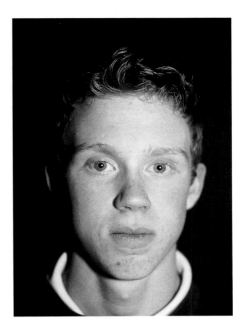
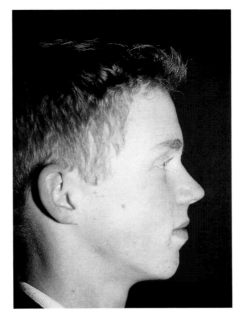

Post treatment

SKELETAL			TEETH		
SNA	°	80.0	Overjet	mm	2.0
SNB	°	77.5	Overbite	mm	2.0
ANB	°	2.5	UI/MxP	°	106.5
SN/MxP	°	2.5	LI/MnP	°	94.0
MxP/MnP	°	34.5	LI-APo	mm	4.5
LAFH/TAFH	%	57.5			

9
Lips can now meet together without difficulty. The lower incisors are now 4.5 mm ahead of A–Po, compared with 8 mm at the start, some residual facial convexity being desirable to preserve the character of the face.

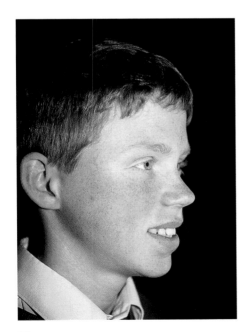
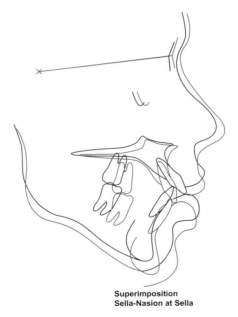
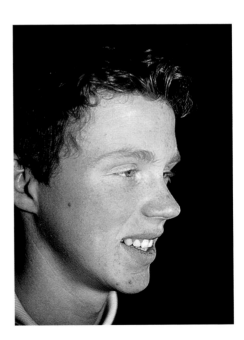

**Superimposition
Sella-Nasion at Sella**

10
Mandibular growth has been reasonably good, with negligible opening of the mandibular angle.

Treatment time = 1 year 7 months.
Routine adjustments = 14.
Archwires used = 6 (3 upper, 3 lower).
Retention = Pre-Fit® (TP Orthondontics Inc., La Porte, Indiana, USA) positioner, followed by upper and lower Hawleys, nights only.

Stage II

Stage II

Objectives

1. **Closure of residual spacing. According to operator choice, this may be either by retraction of labial segments or by protraction of buccal segments.**
2. **Correction of centrelines.**
3. **Derotation of first molars.**
4. **Levelling of first molars.**
5. **Continuing crossbite correction.**
6. **Maintenance of Stage I corrections.**

The second stage is easy to set up and is generally the briefest of the three stages, seldom exceeding 4 months, except perhaps in enforced first molar extraction cases, where there may be relatively large extraction spaces to close. In non-extraction cases, it follows that Stage II may amount to little more than accurate lining up, with .020 inch archwires, prior to the final rectangular Stage III phase.

Timing for Stage II

Irrespective of the starting malocclusion, the second stage should begin synchronously, in both arches, as soon as the first stage objectives have been met. In practice, this means when enamel to enamel contact has been achieved between upper and lower incisors, above the lower incisor brackets. At this time, in a deep bite case, the 'vertical battle' will have been won, so that the anchorage bends can be dispensed with, in favour of conventional vertical 'sweeps' in the archwires, in order to maintain overbite reduction during space closure. In fact, Stage II largely follows straight-wire practice, but with the significant advantage, particularly in extraction cases, that the orthodontist can choose between protractive and retractive mechanics, according to whether or not Side-Winder 'brakes' are placed on the canines.

In all cases, the premolars should be included prior to the start of Stage II.

Aligning the premolars

In cases where the initial overbite was not significantly increased, the premolars will have been bonded from the start of treatment, and will already have been aligned during the first stage. However, in increased overbite cases, where Begg derived mechanics have been used in Stage I, the premolars will have been omitted, and will require to be picked up and aligned at a pre-Stage II visit.

The premolar brackets should be selected with reference to the direction of tooth tip to be accommodated within the bracket, remembering that the second premolar, in a first premolar extraction case, is the exception tooth that comes the opposite way, with mesial crown tip toward the extraction space. A full guide to selection is described in Chapter 6.

The procedure for a deep bite case at the pre-Stage II visit is routine and consists of the following simple steps:

- Remove the .016 inch stainless archwires.
- Bond the premolars.
- Using the same archwires, remove the anchorage bends and replace them with vertical bite sweeps, to retain the overbite reduction previously gained. In the upper arch, this will be an increased curve of Spee, and an inverted curve of Spee in the lower, much as in straight-wire techniques.
- Re-insert the archwires, but into the rectangular molar tubes, which will be used for the remainder of the treatment.

A clinical illustration of the above can be seen by comparing Figure 11.1 with Figure 11.2.

The same .016 inch high tensile stainless archwires, as used throughout Stage I, generally have sufficient flexibility to align the premolars within a 3 week interval. However, there are cases which may require additional help. If a premolar is submerged, for instance, it may not be possible to enter the rectangular molar tube at the pickup visit. It may therefore be necessary to place the archwire in the more gingival round tube, elevating it to the rectangular tube some 2 weeks later.

Another way to deal with wayward premolars is elastic thread, which can be tied through the vertical bracket slots and out to the archwire (Fig. 11.3). This is particularly effective with lingually displaced teeth. Rotated premolars can be corrected with elastomeric E-Links or chain: in the case of a mesial rotation, the elastomeric can run from bracket to molar hook, while a distal rotation will be handled in the

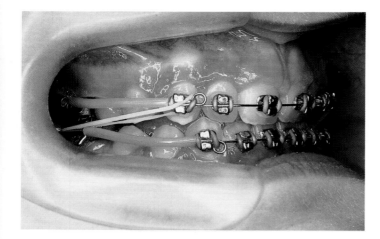

Fig. 11.1 Stage I is complete. It is time to pick up the premolars.

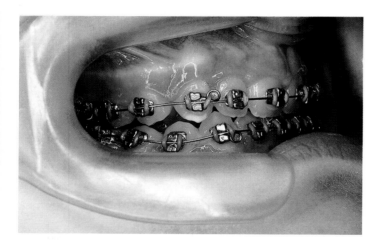

Fig. 11.2 The same archwires now align the premolars to the rectangular molar tubes, bite sweeps replacing the former anchor bends.

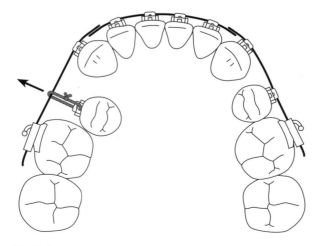

Fig. 11.3 A lingual premolar can be corrected with .020 inch elastic thread.

opposite direction, routing the elastomeric to the cuspid circle (Fig. 11.4). It is seldom necessary to use lingual attachments, although these are a further option for severe rotations.

Just occasionally, we all encounter the awkward premolar that has a combination of problems, being lingually displaced as well as rotated. Although rarely necessary, the nickel-titanium 'underarch' is worth remembering. This can be used sectionally beneath the main archwire if the problem is unilateral (Fig. 11.5A), or one can use a full auxiliary arch,

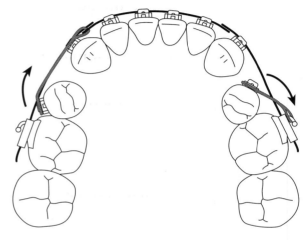

Fig. 11.4 Correction of premolar rotations with elastomeric E-Links: a distal rotation can be linked forward to a cuspid circle (left) and a mesial rotation backwards to a molar hook (right).

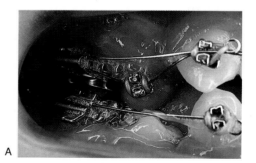

A

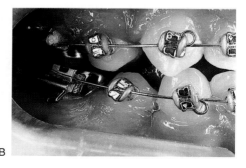

B

Fig. 11.5 (A) A .014 inch nickel-titanium underarch can be used to derotate a lingual rotated premolar to the rectangular molar tube. (B) This correction frequently takes only a month.

worn 'piggy-back' beneath the main archwire. Either way, the premolars need to align to the rectangular molar tubes, the underarch using the rectangular tube and the main arch the round tube. At the following visit, .020 inch archwires should readily engage the rectangular tubes to begin Stage II (Fig. 11.5B). On no account should a nickel-titanium arch be used to align premolars at the end of Stage I without the security of the stainless main arch, as this would invite loss of control elsewhere, such as relapse of overbite and overjet.

Summary of molar tube usage

- Round molar tubes are only used during Stage I in increased overbite cases, when employing Class II elastics and anchorage bends. The premolars will be unbonded.
- As soon as the premolars are bonded, the rectangular tubes are used.
- All subsequent archwires, irrespective of whether round or rectangular, use the rectangular tubes.
- Anchorage and bite opening bends should not be used adjacent to bonded premolars, or in rectangular tubes. In reduced overbite and anterior open bite cases, however, minimal (approximately 5 degrees) molar tip backs are permissible, simply to prevent the molars tipping mesially.

Stage II archwires

As an intermediary wire between the flexible .016 inch stainless first stage archwires and the rigid but passive .0215 × .028 inch rectangular stainless archwires used during the third stage, the author's preference for Stage II is .020 inch high tensile stainless archwires. These are stiff enough to maintain vertical and horizontal control during space closure, but are also sufficiently flexible to allow derotation of the first molars at the end of the stage.

It is however possible to use .022 inch stainless archwires, which will slide through the rectangular molar tubes without undue increase in friction. There may be occasional

indications for using these archwires through Stage II, where the added stiffness (nearly one third greater than .020 inch wires) can be useful:

- In the maxillary arch in crossbite cases, where maxillary buccal segment expansion is required.
- In the mandibular arch in first molar extraction cases, where the heavier archwire offers better labio-lingual control of the second molars and increased resistance to mesial tipping.

Space closure

As in Stage I, the cuspid circles serve as traction hooks. Buccal segment spacing can be closed very easily by applying elastomeric E-Links from the cuspid circles to the molar hooks (Fig. 11.6). Free-sliding mechanics are greatly facilitated throughout Stage II by the design of Tip-Edge brackets, as described in Chapter 3, whereby the binding that causes friction with conventional brackets is eliminated, due to the opening up of the vertical slot dimension during tooth translation. It should also be remembered that the archwire itself will be moving distally, as it travels through the molar tubes.

In addition, the orthodontist is given the choice, when closing buccal segment spacing, between retraction of the labial segment or protraction of the posterior segment, by the simple expedient of adding Side-Winder 'brakes'.

'Applying the brakes'

The principle of 'braking' in variable anchorage has been described in Chapter 2, and is well illustrated in Case 2. Essentially, a gently active Side-Winder can be placed on a canine to induce a distal root movement, anterior to the space to be closed, in each quadrant to be 'braked' (Fig. 11.7). This will significantly increase anterior anchorage, hence resistance to retraction, and so favour protraction of the posterior teeth

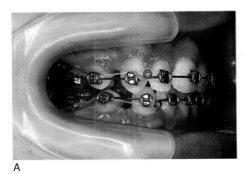
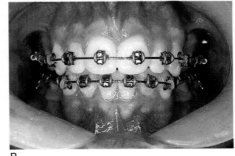
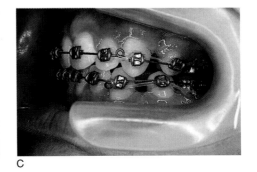

A   B   C

Fig. 11.6 A retractive Stage II set up with .020 inch stainless archwires and E-6 elastomerics to close spaces in all quadrants. This is the same case as shown in Figs 7.1, 7.2 and 7.4, now 8 months into treatment.

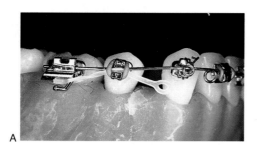

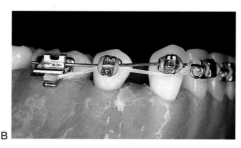

Fig. 11.7 'Braking' on a lower canine. A gently active clockwise Side-Winder (A) will increase anterior anchorage in the lower right quadrant, when hooked up to the archwire (B).

into the space remaining. While the canine is the most common choice as a braked tooth (partly because it offers the largest root area, and also because it frequently requires the most uprighting), a distally inclined first premolar can also be used as a braked unit, as in Case 10.

Braking is frequently used bilaterally, more commonly in the lower arch in Class II cases, and in the upper in Class III cases. Brakes can be applied or removed at any treatment visit, according to the progress of the case. They can also be used unilaterally, as will be seen in the next section, to protect a centreline, or to correct a centreline discrepancy.

Centreline correction

Awareness of centrelines is essential during Stage II, not least because midline discrepancies are most easily corrected while there is still space available in the dental arches. It stands to reason that if the centrelines are not coincident by the time all spaces are closed, there will inevitably be some disparity in the buccal segment occlusion.

Centrelines are more labile with a bracket that allows teeth to tip, but by the same token, they are also much easier to correct. With straight-wire appliances, each anterior unit is essentially a rigidly held 'anchorage unit', requiring to be driven individually to its required position, with appreciable lateral anchorage consequences. By contrast, with Tip-Edge, an entire anterior segment can readily be persuaded to 'flow' laterally into available space, so long as no contrary root resistance is generated.

This frequently works to the clinician's advantage in crowded cases, in which a centreline, if deviated, is almost invariably towards the most crowded side (Fig. 11.8). Such discrepancies may resolve without intervention, for the simple reason that space closure on the worst crowded side will be completed first, whereupon the midline will willingly drift across into the space remaining on the opposite side. However, a watchful eye is required, with a view to placing Side-Winder brakes, usually unilaterally, towards the end of Stage II.

For example, if a centreline is correct at the point where all space has closed on one side but some space remains on the other, a protective brake should be placed on the canine on the spaced side, in order to prevent the labial segment from being pulled across (Fig. 11.9); the remaining space will now be closed by protraction. It follows from this that a centreline cannot be expected to correct if brakes are in action bilaterally (see Case 10).

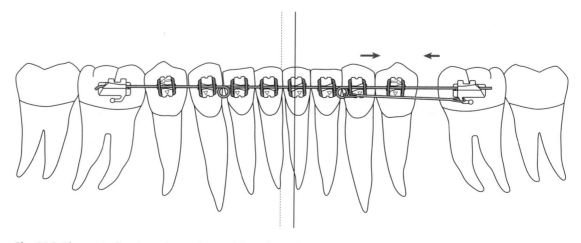

Fig. 11.8 The centreline is to the patient's right, where the extraction space is now closed. Closure of remaining space in the left quadrant will automatically correct the centreline by retraction, without the need for a brake.

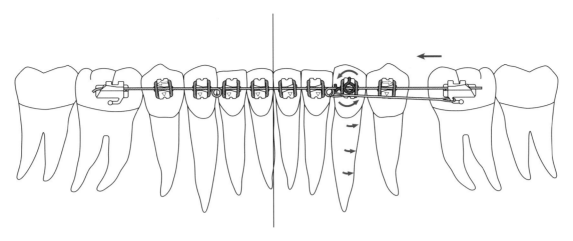

Fig. 11.9 A similar space scenario to Figure 11.8, but with a correct centreline. A defensive brake is now required to the left canine, so that the remaining unilateral space is closed by protraction, thus preserving the centreline.

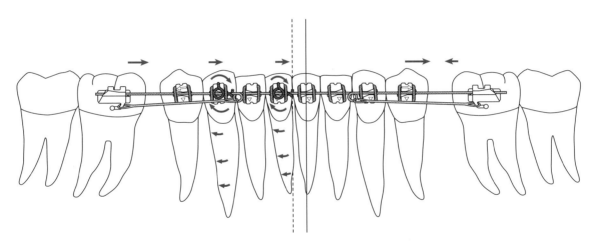

Fig. 11.10 Active correction of a centreline. Here, space exists in both quadrants, and the centreline needs correcting into the patient's left quadrant space, by retraction, whereas the space remaining in the right quadrant must be closed by protraction. The lower right canine is therefore braked. In this illustration, an additional Side-Winder is placed on the right central incisor, for distal root movement, thereby helping the centreline across.

It is also possible to influence centrelines from the front of the arch. Applying a Side-Winder to a mesially tipped central, or even a lateral, incisor will induce a lateral movement across the segment and influence the centreline movement towards the opposite side, particularly if supplemented by a brake to the canine behind it (Fig. 11.10).

Inevitably, centreline corrections in non-extraction cases may be more challenging, as with any technique, particularly if no arch space is available. This frequently denotes an underlying skeletal component. As with straight-wire, possible options may be unilateral intermaxillary elastics, or anterior transverse elastics. In either scenario, with free-tipping brackets during Stage II, Tip-Edge will prove more responsive to lighter forces than conventional bracket systems.

Derotation of first molars

During Stage II, a limited amount of first molar rotation can be expected as a result of space closure with free-sliding mechanics. This is simply because the archwire of .020 inch diameter runs within a molar tube of .028 inch lateral dimension, so that active space closure will express this freeplay as mesial rotation, as the molar slides along the wire. It is a mistake to try and prevent this from happening, as placement of buccal offsets and toe-ins adds friction to the

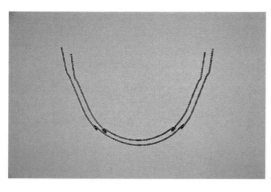

Fig. 11.11 One millimetre molar offsets and 10 degrees of toe-in for final visit of Stage II (.020 inch archwire).

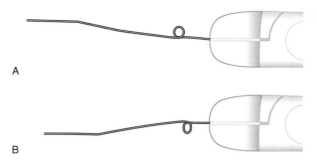

A

B

Fig. 11.12 Anti-tip bends in .020 inch wire ensure seating of the distal cusps of tipped molars at the conclusion of Stage II. These can be combined with the offset and toe-in placed at the same visit.

process, and need regular repositioning. It is much better, therefore, to allow the molars to slide along the wire unhindered. Only at the final visit of Stage II, when space is closed, should the molars be derotated.

This requires a simple adjustment to the archwire, placing a 1 mm buccal offset and 10 degrees of lingual toe-in opposite the interspace between the first molar and premolar (Fig. 11.11). To prevent space recurring, the distal archwire ends should be annealed and turned gingivally.

Normally, it takes only 3 weeks to derotate first molars. However, it is of paramount importance that this simple step should not be omitted. It stands to reason that while a small amount of mesial molar rotation will not interfere with the insertion of a .020 inch wire, it only takes a very small amount of mesial rotation to completely obstruct a .028 inch lateral dimension rectangular wire, which virtually fills the tube. Forgetting to derotate the molars at the end of Stage II is the commonest reason for difficulty in fitting rectangular wires at the following visit.

Levelling of first molars

In deep bite cases treated with Class II elastics and anchor bends, it is not uncommon for some distal crown tipping of the first molars to have occurred, since the roots will have been inclined mesially, to boost anchorage resistance throughout Stage I. Obviously, as anchor bends are not used in the second stage, there will be a natural tendency for molar angulations to correct anyway, and more so in an extraction case, where mesial migration into the extraction space will itself tend to eliminate any distal crown tip. However, in a non-extraction case, first molars that have been worked hard during overbite and overjet reduction may need positive correction during the brief Stage II.

The vertical adjustment in the archwire can be combined with the molar derotation adjustment, opposite the premolar to molar contact point. It consists essentially of an 'anti-tip' bend of no more than 10 degrees, aimed at seating the distal

molar cusps into occlusion (Fig. 11.12). In a Stage II .020 stainless wire, untipping of molars can frequently be effected in a single short visit. It is essential that the molar tubes are lined up horizontal and level with the brackets, as the heavier gauge rectangular archwires, shortly to follow, will not accommodate vertical discrepancies.

Continuing crossbite correction

Buccal segment expansion is naturally more effective during second stage than with the lighter Stage I archwires. As already mentioned, there may be a case for using the heavier .022 inch archwire option in the maxilla, to gain more effective expansion. Either way, it is desirable to complete crossbite correction by the end of Stage II if possible since, although the rectangular wires of third stage have impressive expansion potential (particularly if torque assisted), this will usually entail archwire removal at some point during Stage III, which should not otherwise be necessary.

Maintenance of Stage I corrections

This is chiefly a matter of preserving the incisor relationship, gained during Stage I, throughout the second stage. The aim is to keep the enamel to enamel contact between upper and lower incisors at the midline. A patient can be taught to recognize this, and should be instructed to maintain this light contact by regulating the traction accordingly. With experience, the operator can assess any likely effect Stage II may have on the interarch relationship, depending on which arch spaces are to be closed and whether or not brakes are in use. Mandibular growth is another influencing factor. Therefore, if Class II elastics are the anchorage source, the patient will need to wear these as much as is needed to maintain the incisor relationship. In practice, nights only wear, or perhaps evenings and nights, is the likely expectation; it is unusual for full time elastic wear to be necessary once beyond Stage I. Likewise, if a patient is a headgear wearer, this will require to be worn for as many nights a week as proves necessary to keep incisor contact.

CASE 5

A deep bite Class II division 2 malocclusion with mild crowding

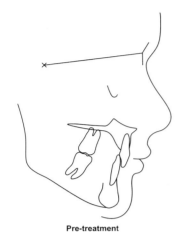

Pre-treatment

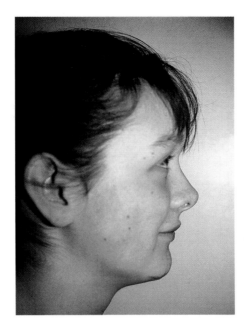
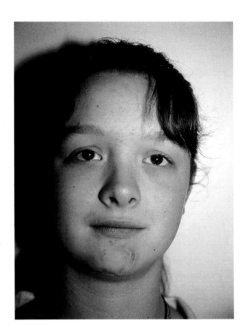

SKELETAL			TEETH			
SNA	°	75.0	Overjet	mm	4.5
SNB	°	72.0	Overbite	mm	7.5
ANB	°	3.0	UI/MxP	°	86.0
SN/MxP	°	11.0	LI/MnP	°	76.0
MxP/MnP	°	25.0	LI-APo	mm	-5.5
LAFH/TAFH	%	51.5			

1
A mild skeletal Class II case with a reduced MM angle (25 degrees) and a significantly reduced lower face height (51.5%). At 15 years 8 months, the patient is older than is ideally suited to this procedure, with little growth remaining. The lower incisors are 5.5 mm behind the A–Po line.

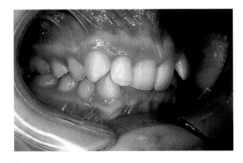
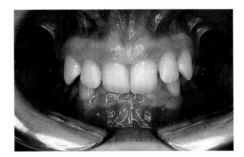
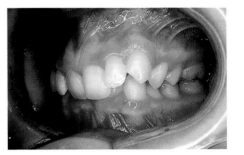

2
Both upper and lower anterior segments are typically retroclined, with an increased overbite which threatens to become traumatic. There is mild crowding of incisors and canines in both arches.

Premolar extractions are contraindicated, but upper second molars will be extracted to accommodate the unerupted wisdom teeth.

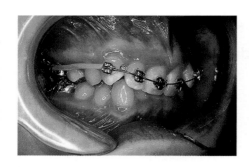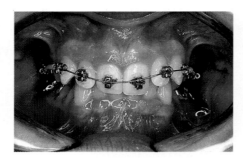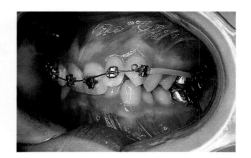

3

It is good practice to procline the upper incisors away from the lowers in the initial treatment visit. This avoids the risk of bite damage to the lower incisor brackets, and also prevents the extrusion of opposed first molars if temporarily out of occlusion due to anterior bracket interference. Here, a .016 inch high tensile stainless upper archwire is used, loose tied to the upper central incisors, with buccal sleeves and light tip back bends in the first molars.

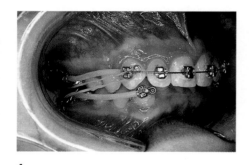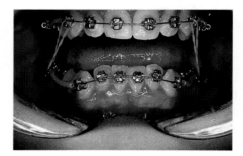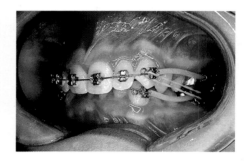

4

At the following visit, Stage I begins. The lower arch is included without bite interference. Anchor bends immediately mesial to all molar round tubes begin overbite reduction, in combination with 50 grams Class II full time elastics, buccal sleeves preventing premolar crowding. The open view shows that the lingual lower lateral incisors are tied with .020 inch elastomeric thread through the vertical slots.

Another reason for proclining upper incisors prior to Stage I is that intrusion of a normally angulated or proclined upper incisor will result in a favourable palatal root path, whereas intruding a retroclined incisor may drive the apex further labially, adding to the amount of torque that will later be required.

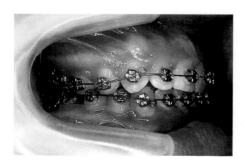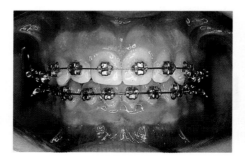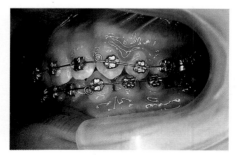

5

Bite planes are not required to assist overbite reduction with Tip-Edge. The overbite reduces irrespective of canine angulation, and 9 months into treatment opposing incisors are contacting above the lower brackets and the occlusion has translated to Class I. The premolars are included and aligned with the existing archwires, bite sweeps replacing the anchorage bends and the rectangular tubes will be used throughout the remainder of treatment. Intermaxillary elastics will need to be worn only part time, sufficient to retain the new interarch relationship.

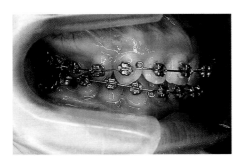
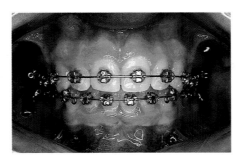
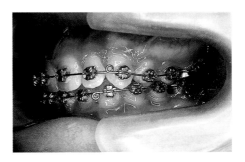

6

Interim .020 inch swept stainless archwires are worn for only a single visit, to level and derotate the first molars with offsets and toe-ins.

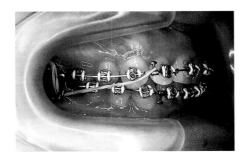
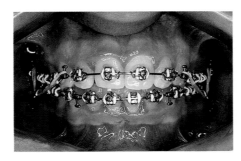
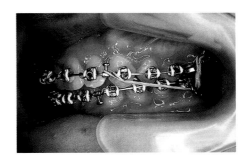

7

Pretorqued .0215 × .028 inch archwires are selected, since vertical bite sweeps will be required to maintain overbite reduction. The pretorque will neutralize the labial crown torque to the incisors, which would otherwise result from the bite sweeps. However, in Class II division 2 cases, some additional bite sweep to the maxillary archwire, compared to normal, can be used to advantage. If a normal sweep amounts to zero torque, an increased sweep will produce a small amount of extra torque, over the Rx-1 torque in base prescription, thereby overcorrecting the interincisal angle.

The Class II 'check' elastics, worn at nights, are sometimes helpful to maintain molar approximation.

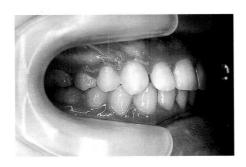
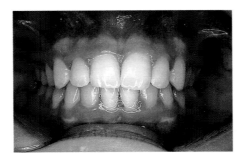
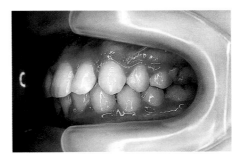

8

After 6 months in Stage III, treatment is complete, with torque and tip achieved for each tooth individually, and with some additional torque to the upper incisors.

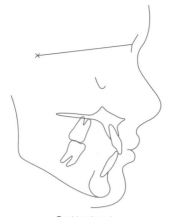

Post treatment

SKELETAL			TEETH		
SNA	°	73.0	Overjet	mm	2.5
SNB	°	73.0	Overbite	mm	1.5
ANB	°	0.5	UI/MxP	°	113.0
SN/MxP	°	11.5	LI/MnP	°	94.0
MxP/MnP	°	24.5	LI-APo	mm	2.0
LAFH/TAFH	%	51.5			

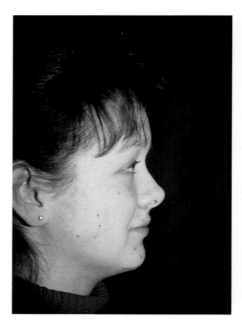

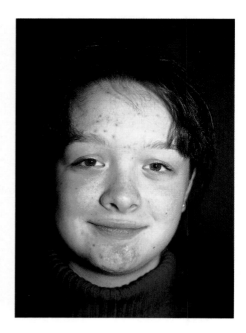

9
Labial advancement of the dentition has greatly enhanced facial fullness. The lower incisors lie 2 mm ahead of A–Po.

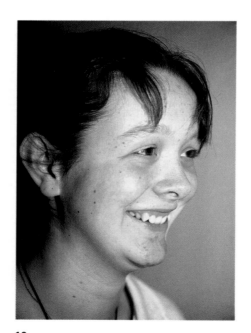

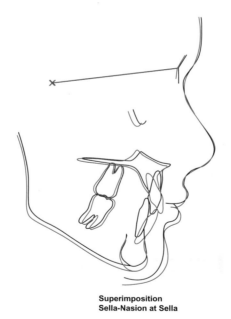

**Superimposition
Sella-Nasion at Sella**

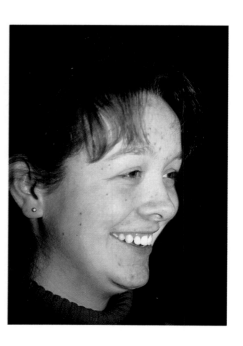

10
Growth has been predictably little in extent, and the lower labial segment will require lingual bonded retention. A considerable improvement in gummy smile is evident facially.

Treatment time = 1 year 8 months.
Routine adjustments = 12.
Archwires used = 6 (3 upper, 3 lower).
Retention = upper Hawleys, nights only, lower lingual bonded retainer.

CASE 6

A severely crowded Class II division 2 malocclusion on a marked skeletal II base

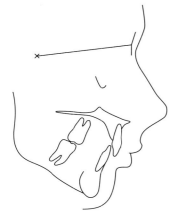

Pre-treatment

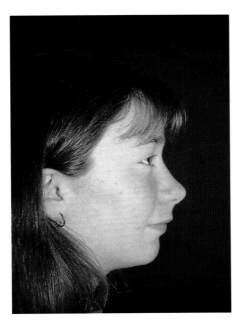

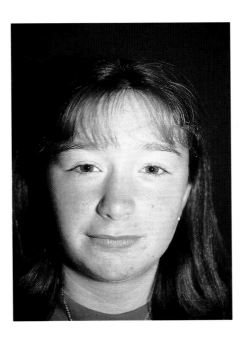

SKELETAL			TEETH		
SNA	°	76.5	Overjet	mm	5.0
SNB	°	70.0	Overbite	mm	6.0
ANB	°	6.5	UI/MxP	°	88.5
SN/MxP	°	15.0	LI/MnP	°	86.0
MxP/MnP	°	25.5	LI-APo	mm	-3.0
LAFH/TAFH	%	51.0			

1
At 14 years 4 months, a challenging case! An ANB angle of 6.5 degrees confirms an appreciable Class II skeletal discrepancy, with a reduction in lower face height (51%) and maxillary mandibular planes angle (25.5 degrees). The upper central incisors are severely retroclined and the lower incisors lie 3 mm behind A–Po. Skeletally, the case is suitable for Class II intermaxillary traction.

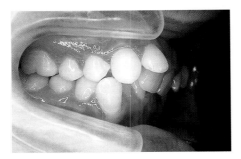

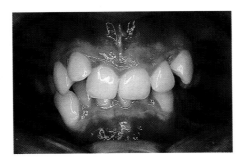

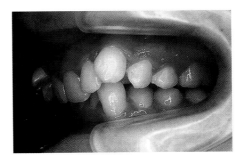

2
The overbite is increased and complete and both arches are severely crowded anteriorly. The lower right canine has a particularly adverse inclination. The buccal segment occlusion is a full unit Class II on the right, and is little better on the left. This degree of crowding necessitates premolar extractions. In consideration of the retrusive profile, four second premolars were preferred to first premolar extractions.

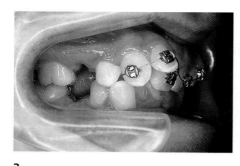
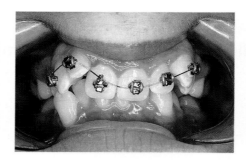
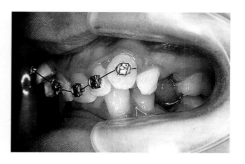

3

For the same reasons as in Case 5, prior proclination of the upper incisors is indicated before bonding the lower arch. In this case, the incisor displacements are too extreme to allow comfortable use of a stainless archwire. Consequently, preliminary alignment involves a sectional .012 inch nickel-titanium wire. To avoid loss of extraction space in this maximum discrepancy case, rapid progression to stainless archwires with anchor bends must be planned.

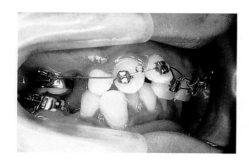
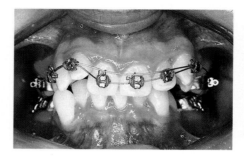
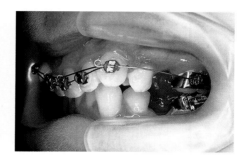

4

Three weeks later, it is possible to supplement the sectional with a .016 inch high tensile stainless archwire, loose tied into the upper central incisors. Light tip-back bends prevent mesial drifting of the upper molars.

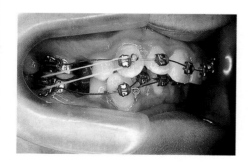
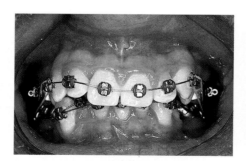
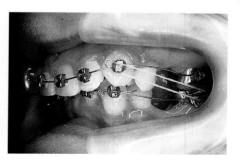

5

At the following visit Stage I begins. The upper arch can be fully engaged, with cuspid circles rolled distally, and a matching lower arch is fitted with a .012 inch nickel-titanium underarch to align the instanding incisors. Strong anchor bends are employed to all round first molar tubes, in combination with 50 grams Class II elastics. In common with previous increased overbite cases, the premolars are omitted until overbite reduction is complete.

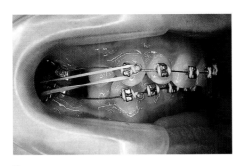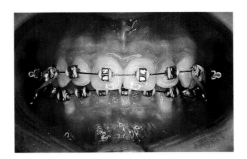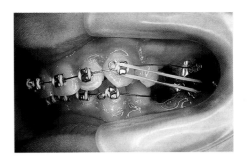

6
Three months later, the lower anteriors are aligned, so the underarch can be discarded. Reduction of overbite and overjet are ongoing.

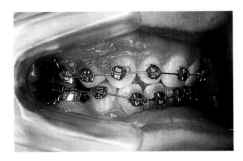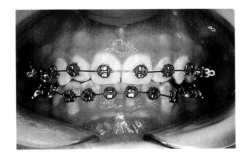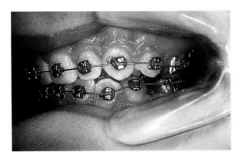

7
Incisor contact has been achieved above the lower incisor brackets. The premolars are therefore bonded, for alignment to the rectangular molar tubes, using the existing archwires but with bite sweeps replacing the anchor bends. As with previous cases, the round molar tubes will not be used again and night time elastic wear will normally be enough to retain the new incisor relationship throughout remaining treatment.

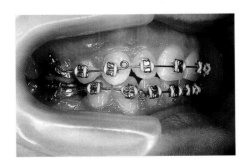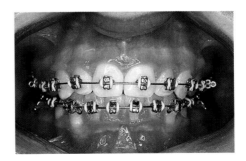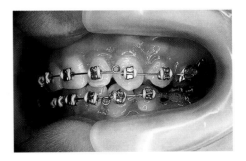

8
Only lower extraction spaces remain. With swept .020 inch Stage II stainless archwires, Side-Winder brakes are added to both lower canines. The E-5 elastomeric intramaxillary links will therefore protract the lower molars towards a Class I relationship.

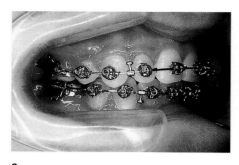
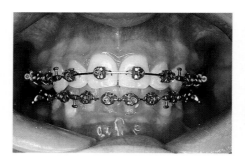
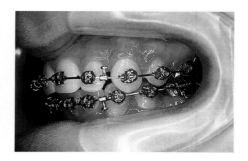

9

Stage III .0215 × .028 inch pretorqued archwires are similar in set up to Case 5. The lower archwire has been swept to a zero torque setting across the incisor segment, while the upper is slightly 'overswept' past the zero torque position, to produce some additional torque and overbite control. Elastic wear will normally be nights only, to maintain the interarch fit, although this may vary between different individuals according to mandibular growth.

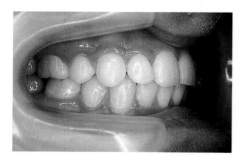
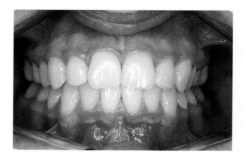
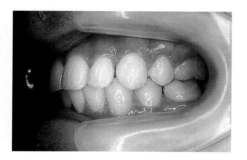

10

Torque and tip have been fully expressed for all bracketed teeth individually by the Side-Winders.

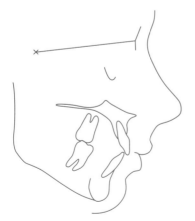

Post treatment

SKELETAL			TEETH		
SNA	°	75.5	Overjet	mm	3.0
SNB	°	72.0	Overbite	mm	1.0
ANB	°	3.5	UI/MxP	°	114.0
SN/MxP	°	14.5	LI/MnP	°	101.0
MxP/MnP	°	22.0	LI-APo	mm	2.5
LAFH/TAFH	%	52.0			

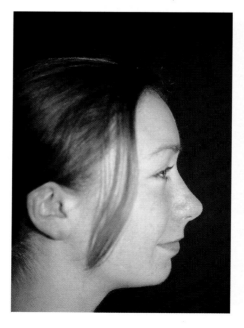
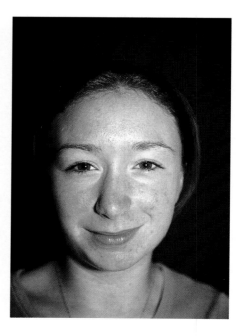

11

The interincisal angle has been overcorrected with a much improved facial profile.

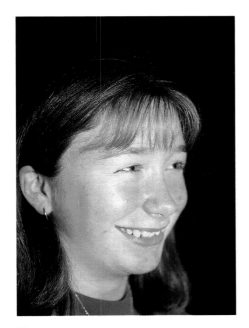
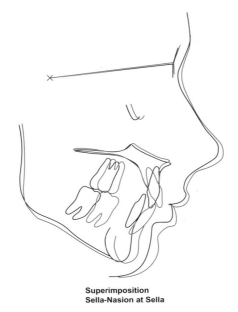
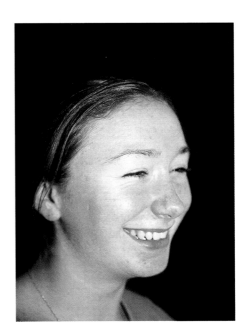

**Superimposition
Sella-Nasion at Sella**

12
Mandibular growth has been good, with no opening of the mandibular angle. The skeletal pattern has therefore improved (ANB reduced by 3 degrees) and there is also an improvement in gummy smile.

Treatment time = 1 year 11 months.
Routine adjustments = 16.
Archwires used = 6 (3 upper, 3 lower).
Retention = upper and lower Hawleys, nights only.

Setting up Stage II

Setting up Stage II

Stage II is very easy to set up and maintain, and has much in common with straight-wire practice.

Archwire preparation

Preformed arches are available and represent a considerable time saving. Made from .020 (or .022) inch Bow-Flex high tensile stainless steel, selection is similar to that described for Stage I, using the intraoral measure to determine the desired distance between the cuspid circles. However, in Stage II, the cuspid circles require to be somewhat further mesially from the canine brackets (Fig. 12.1). This is so as not to obstruct the possible placement of brakes on the canines, when the arms of the Side-Winders will point mesially. Mid-way between the canine and lateral incisor brackets is therefore the best place for the cuspid circles. The position of these circles will not require any subsequent adjustment.

Archform will be essentially similar to Stage I, with the anterior curvature extending distal to the canines (Fig. 12.2). However, there will be no anchor bends, and there is no need to incorporate any expansion unless, of course, a crossbite is being corrected. A straight posterior leg is preferred down the buccal segments, as this avoids the complex double curvature when combining a vertical bite sweep with a buccal convexity.

The archwire can readily be tailored for arch width and length, leaving 2 mm projecting distal to each molar tube. These ends can be annealed.

Whether or not vertical bite sweeps will be required will depend on the initial degree of overbite. If the overbite was originally decreased, the archwires can be fitted flat, whereas a case that started with an increased overbite will need bite sweeps, in order to retain the overbite reduction gained

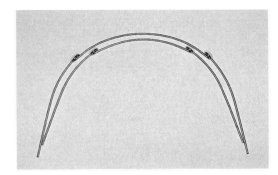

Fig. 12.2 Stage II archform (.020 inch archwires).

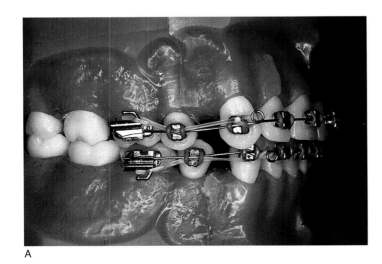

A

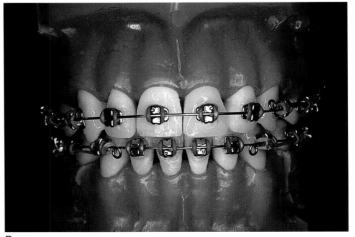

B

Fig. 12.1 Stage II with .020 inch archwires.

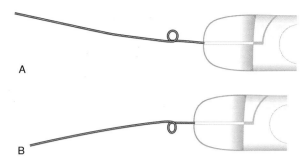

Fig. 12.3 Vertical 'bite sweeps' will be needed to maintain a previously reduced overbite.

during the first stage. These will consist of a reverse curve of Spee in the lower arch and an increased curve of Spee, or 'rocking horse' curve, in the upper (Fig. 12.3).

Wiping in the vertical sweeps is best done with thumb and finger while holding the archwire immediately distal to the circle in a light wire plier. A mistake commonly made is to wipe in the sweeps before cutting the distal arch ends to length, in which case the operator has less idea of precisely what length of sweep is relevant to the mouth. This also introduces the danger of extending the sweeps into the molar tubes, which will tend to perpetuate distal crown tip of the molars. Vertical bite curvatures work best when confined to the canine and premolar regions.

As for the angle of sweep, this is readily estimated on insertion. Between a millimetre or two of active intrusion in the archwire will generally be sufficient to retain a reduced overbite, as measured at the midline.

Fitting the arches

Rectangular molar tubes are invariably used throughout Stage II. All six upper and lower anterior brackets are ligated with elastomerics in the usual way.

Space closure is carried out using elastomeric E-Links. These are preferred to elastomeric chain, the force of which can only be crudely adjusted according to the number of links chosen. E-Links come in graded lengths (Fig. 12.4) and clinical experience suggests a respectable working life of up to 3 months in the mouth, although they will normally be replaced at 6-weekly intervals.

Each E-link runs from the buccal hook on the first molar to the cuspid circle. In a premolar extraction case, an E6 will most often be the appropriate size, sometimes progressing to an E5 when the space has almost closed. It will be noted that in sizes E5 and above, a small tail is provided,* but this is not relevant to Stage II. Either the tail can be amputated with ligature cutters, or placed at the distal end of the link, where it

---

*This enables the E-link to be used as a lassoo, by feeding the tail through the circle at the opposite end and pulling tight. This may occasionally be useful for retrieving impacted teeth early in treatment.

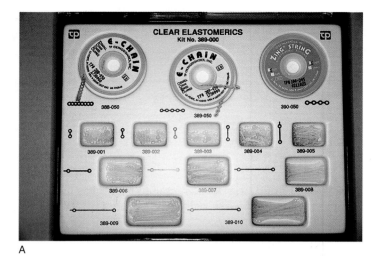

A

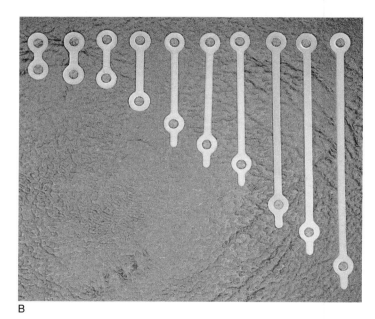

B

Fig. 12.4 E-Links come in 10 available sizes.

will be concealed behind the molar hook and will not worry the patient.

Because the mesial end of the E-link is attached to the cuspid circle, it is not necessary to ligate the canine brackets to the cuspid circles as well, either during Stage II, or at any future time in treatment. The reason is that the E-Links exert an overall space-condensing force from the cuspid circles, which will also prevent the archwire sliding from side to side.

A long strand of elastomeric running parallel to the archwire may constitute a 'fiddle factor' for the patient, which is why the author prefers to route the E-Link beneath the retaining module on the premolar. This makes it less conspicuous. The sequence of placement is illustrated in Figure 12.5.

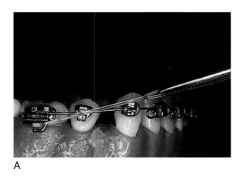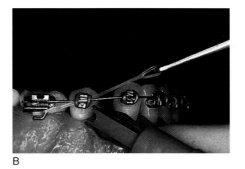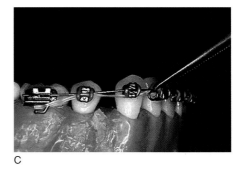

A   B   C

Fig. 12.5 Placement of E-Links. (A) The operator engages the molar hook and stretches the E-link across the premolar bracket. (B) The assistant holds the E-link in position while the operator ligatures the premolar. (C) The operator engages the forward end around the cuspid circle.

The arch ends can be annealed and bent lingually, distal to the molar tubes, to preserve patient comfort as the ends grow longer, during space closure. However, if the space has already closed, this can be retained by cinching the arch end gingivally.

Care should be taken in Stage II not to over close spaces, by provoking overlapping contacts. Not only can this encourage relapse of previous rotations but, as will be stressed in Stage III, teeth require additional mesio-distal space when being uprighted. Tight contacts will 'choke' the action of the Side-Winders during the third stage, and is one of the major reasons for inadequate expression of final torque and tip angles.

Adding brakes

If a quadrant is to be braked, a Side-Winder auxiliary spring will be required, usually to the canine, but possibly to a first premolar, or even to both. Using invisible Side-Winders, the spring should be inserted down the vertical slot from the occlusal before placing the elastomeric ligature. The arm of each spring, when used as a brake, should point mesially (Fig. 12.6). Activation of the spring should not normally exceed 45 degrees for braking purposes.

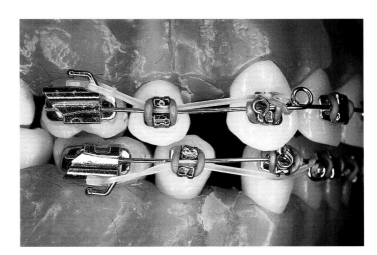

Fig. 12.6 Brakes placed on upper and lower canines for a 'protractive' Stage II.

Stage II checks

Stage II checks

The routine adjustment interval in Stage II is 6 weeks, but can sometimes be extended to 8 weeks. It is not normally necessary to remove the archwires, except at or towards the end of the stage, when offsets and toe-ins will need to be placed, to derotate the first molars.

At each adjustment visit, the following checks will be necessary:

- **Observe space closure.** This can either be measured direct, or gauged by the amount of excess archwire protruding from the distal of the molar tubes. Where further space remains to be closed, the elastomeric E-Links should be replaced. *Obstruction to space closure is rare, but can be caused by premature placement of toe-ins to the first molars.*

- **The distal archwire ends.** These should be trimmed back to 2 mm of distal projection and turned slightly to the lingual, for the comfort of the patient. If all space has closed in a particular quadrant, the respective distal archwire end should be annealed and turned gingivally, to prevent the space reopening.

- **Check molar widths.** Normally, these will not require adjustment, unless a crossbite is being corrected.

- **Labial segment position and inclination.** This may require the addition or removal of brakes, according to whether remaining space closure is required by retraction of the incisors, or by protraction of the molars. *Excessive retroclination of upper incisors should be avoided (by placement of brakes on upper canines), as this may encourage apical resorption.*

- **Attention to centrelines.** Except in the case of big midline discrepancies, remedial action will not be required until towards the end of the second stage. At that time, the application of selective brakes should be considered, as described in Chapter 11, usually unilaterally. This may be to induce active centreline correction (see Fig. 11.10) or to defend against an unwanted late shift (see Fig. 11.9) when space remains on one side but not on the other. *Failure to obtain coincident midlines by the end of Stage II will inevitably result in an occlusal discrepancy, which will be less easy to correct in Stage III.*

- **Derotation of first molars.** Only relevant at the end of Stage II, this is essential once the space has closed. A 1 mm buccal offset and 10 degrees of lingual toe-in should be added to the archwire at the molar–premolar interspace, as outlined in Chapter 11. *Failure to do this will make it difficult or impossible to enter the molar tubes with rectangular archwires at the next visit.*

- **'Un-tip' the first molars.** Of likely relevance to deep bite non-extraction cases, where Begg-derived mechanics have been used during Stage I, anti-tip bends may be required to seat the disto-buccal cusps, as described in Chapter 11. *Again, it will be difficult or impossible to feed a rectangular archwire into a distally tipped molar at the Stage III visit.*

- **Avoid overcompression.** At the end of space closure, tight or overlapping contacts should be relieved, by relaxing the gingival cinchbacks at the distal arch ends. *Contact point pressure will significantly retard or halt correction of torque and tip in the following stage.*

- **Check the interarch relationship.** Is the patient observing and maintaining their incisor relationship as instructed? Is the intermaxillary traction (or headgear) being worn sufficiently to maintain Stage I corrections?

A Class I case with anterior crowding

Case 7 introduces Tip-Edge in a different context and in a more conventional mode. All cases described hitherto have been Class II malocclusions. Because the initial overbites needed reduction, in patients not exhibiting a significant increase in lower facial height, the anchorage source chosen has been Class II intermaxillary elastics with first molar anchorage bends. The reason for this source of anchorage, which is preferred in Class II cases when possible, is simply convenience and ease of cooperation for the patient (compared with addition of headgear, for example).

In a Class I malocclusion, however, interarch correction of the incisors will not be necessary, and without the interarch component, anchorage will normally be less demanding. The commonest objectives are decrowding and alignment, for which anchorage may frequently be obtained from within each arch, particularly if it is an extraction case.

In Case 7, all anchorage is derived intra-arch. Bodily control of the first molars within conventional rectangular molar tubes is pitted against free tipping of the anterior teeth during the unravelling process. Having said which, traction of any kind is frequently unnecessary in Stage I. The anterior

unravelling results from a freewheeling process of distal canine drifting, in response to a light nickel titanium archwire aligning the lateral incisors. The molars merely maintain their position, or drift a little mesially. This can be seen in the maxillary arch of Case 7. The lower arch is treated differently but only because of a suspected Class III tendency. A nickel titanium under arch beneath a stainless .016 inch main archwire in conjunction with Class III elastic traction would be a legitimate alternative, but this would necessitate an upper stainless archwire also, to support the elastics. Overall, the method illustrated is simpler both for operator and the patient. Without recourse to Class III elastics, the lower canines are retracted gently along the archwire, just as in straight wire, delaying alignment of the instanding lateral incisors until space is available. This small precaution ensures against precipitating a reverse overjet.

It should be noted that, as always, the progression and sequence of the three stages stays the same, whatever the malocclusion type, even though the means of achieving each stage (particularly Stage I) and the anchorage source may differ.

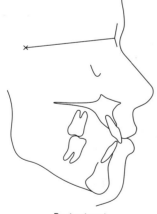

Pre-treatment

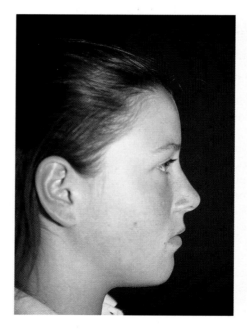 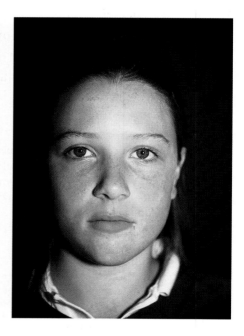

SKELETAL			TEETH		
SNA	°	82.5	Overjet	mm	3.0
SNB	°	81.0	Overbite	mm	0.5
ANB	°	1.5	UI/MxP	°	117.5
SN/MxP	°	6.5	LI/MnP	°	99.0
MxP/MnP	°	26.5	LI-APo	mm	4.0
LAFH/TAFH	%	58.0			

1
At 14 years 11 months, a relatively normal skeletal pattern, although there is a mild Class III tendency suggested by a reduction in overbite and overjet. Although the mandibular–maxillary planes angle is within normal limits, lower face height is increased (58%). Here is an example of treatment with horizontal mechanics and anchorage along edgewise lines, while incorporating the advantages of differential tooth movement. Since no overbite reduction will be required, round molar tubes are omitted and the premolars will be bonded from the outset.

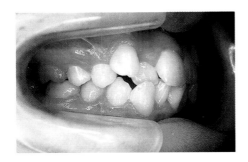
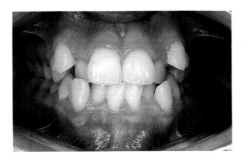
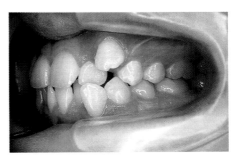

2
All four lateral incisors are bodily displaced lingually, of which the uppers are in reverse overjet. The upper canines are severely crowded and the lower right canine is distally inclined.

Since the profile is fully procumbent (lower incisors 4 mm in front of A–Po), four premolar extractions will be indicated to accommodate the crowding. Taking account of a possible underlying Class III growth pattern, the extractions chosen are upper second and lower first premolars.

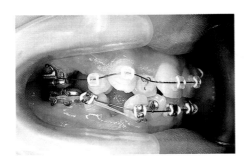
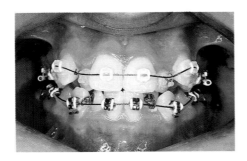
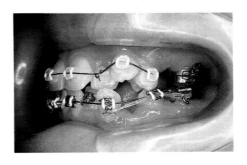

3
Stage I begins with an upper .014 inch nickel-titanium archwire, loose tied into the lateral incisors. This may tend to advance the upper anterior teeth slightly. In a potential Class III situation, however, the same must be avoided in the lower, in order to guard against reversing the overjet. The lower canines are therefore first retracted along a .016 inch stainless archwire, which is stopped mesial to the lower first molars to conserve available extraction space. The lower lateral incisors have passive loose ties, the right lateral carrying a loop until a bracket can be correctly placed. Note that the E-6 elastomeric links attach to Power Pins on the canines, instead of directly to the brackets, to avoid distal rotation.

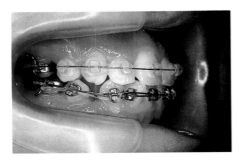
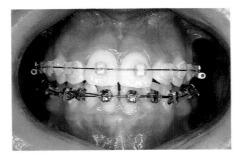
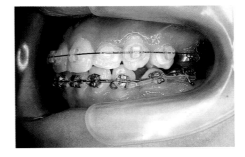

4
At the first adjustment visit, the upper arch is already levelled and aligned, and the lower canines have tipped distally enough for placement of a correct bracket on the rotated right lateral. The stopped lower arch is replaced with a free sliding .016 inch stainless archwire and the E-Links (E-5) are now applied to the cuspid circles for intramaxillary traction, while a .014 inch nickel-titanium underarch is tied tightly into the right lateral incisor for derotation.

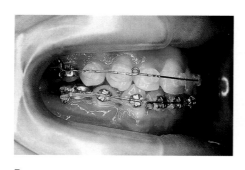
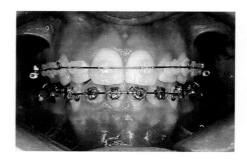
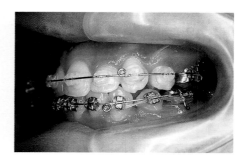

5

Level .020 inch stainless Stage II archwires are fitted. All upper extraction space has closed by itself along the original nickel-titanium archwire. A small amount of lower extraction space requires to be closed by horizontal E-5 elastomerics. A Side-Winder to the lower left central incisor protects the lower centreline.

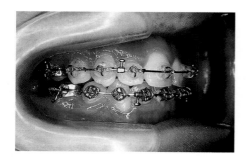
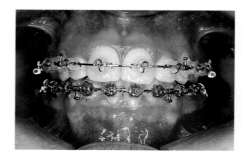
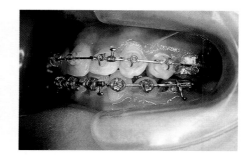

6

At the following visit, Stage III .0215 × 028 inch rectangular archwires are fitted. No bite sweeps will be used at any time during treatment, so flat zero torque archwires can be fitted without any torque adjustment. Note the present torque discrepancies between the upper central and lateral incisors.

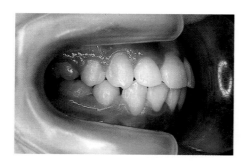
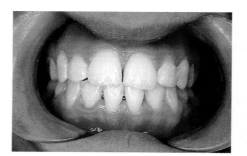
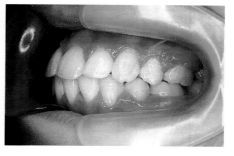

7

After 8 months, the Side-Winders have expressed the torque and tip for each bracketed tooth individually. Mechanics have been horizontal intramaxillary throughout, with no intermaxillary elastics. Inverted brackets were *not* required on the upper lateral incisors, for reasons explained in Chapter 14.

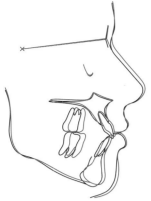

**Superimposition
Sella-Nasion at Sella**

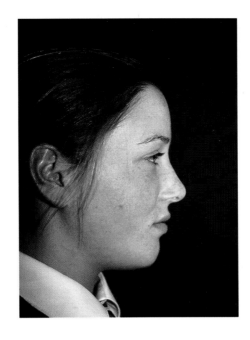

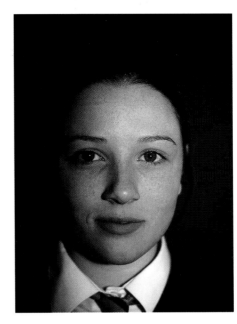

SKELETAL			TEETH		
SNA	°	82.0	Overjet	mm	2.0
SNB	°	81.5	Overbite	mm	2.0
ANB	°	1.0	UI/MxP	°	121.5
SN/MxP	°	8.0	LI/MnP	°	98.5
MxP/MnP	°	23.5	LI-APo	mm	5.0
LAFH/TAFH	%	57.5			

8
The profile has been well preserved. In the event, little further mandibular growth has taken place and the skeletal pattern has scarcely deteriorated.

Treatment time = 1 year 4 months.
Routine adjustments = 10.
Archwires used = 7 (3 upper, 4 lower).
Retention = upper and lower Hawleys, nights only.

A Class III case with a complex reverse overjet

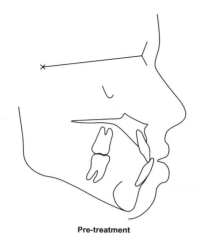

Pre-treatment

SKELETAL			TEETH		
SNA	°	85.0	Overjet	mm	-3.0
SNB	°	83.0	Overbite	mm	3.0
ANB	°	2.0	UI/MxP	°	110.5
SN/MxP	°	9.0	LI/MnP	°	96.5
MxP/MnP	°	23.0	LI-APo	mm	7.5
LAFH/TAFH	%	56.0			

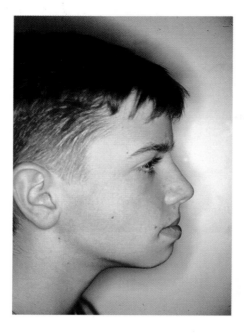

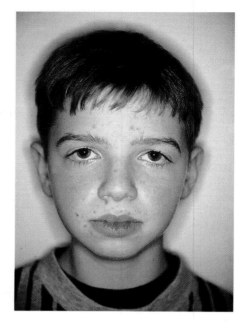

1

A skeletal Class III case at 13 years 10 months, with a slight reduction in maxillary–mandibular planes angle (23 degrees). The crowded lower central incisors are procumbent, suggesting that some retraction should be possible to enable a positive overjet correction. As in Case 7, horizontal mechanics will be used throughout treatment, since overbite reduction will not be required. Round molar tubes will not be necessary and the premolars will be included from the beginning.

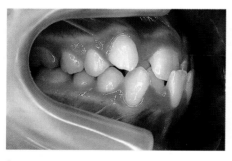

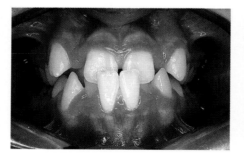

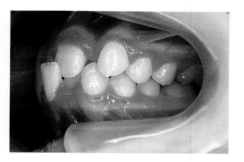

2

Described by the parent as 'four rows of teeth', this is a bizarre pattern of incisor crowding and reverse overjet interlock, surprisingly without forward mandibular displacement. All four lateral incisors are bodily displaced lingually, the uppers grossly.

Since the lower central incisors are 8 mm in front of A–Po and both anterior segments are considerably crowded, four premolar extractions will be indicated. These will be lower first premolars, to accommodate the crowding and lingual repositioning, but upper first premolars are retained to help support a proclined upper incisor segment in positive overjet, second premolar extractions being preferred.

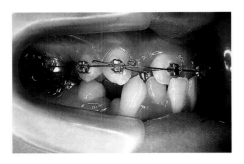
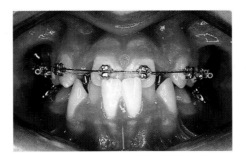
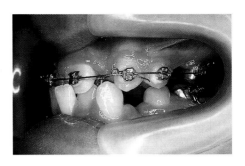

3

Anterior bite interference prevents bracketing of the lower lateral incisors initially. The reverse overjet is therefore tackled in two stages, upper arch first. A .016 inch high tensile stainless archwire is fitted flat. The upper lateral incisors carry temporary brackets, into which a .012 inch nickel-titanium underarch is loosely tied.

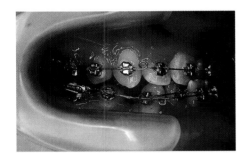
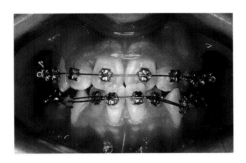
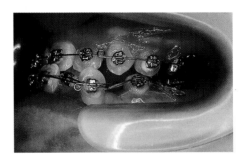

4

Three months later, the upper laterals are in positive overjet and can be correctly bracketed. The underarch is discarded. Much of the upper extraction space has closed by distal drifting of the canines and premolars.

Lower arch treatment begins with a flat .016 inch high tensile stainless archwire with a .014 inch nickel-titanium underarch to align the instanding lower lateral incisors. Intramaxillary traction with E-5 elastomerics will correct the reverse overjet on the lower central incisors.

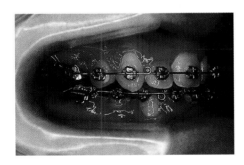
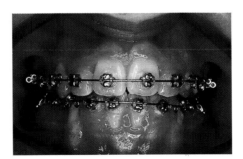
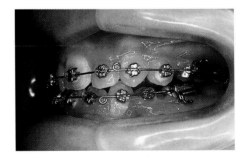

5

The objectives of Stage I are essentially the same in Class III cases as for other malocclusion types, and have been achieved in 8 months.

Since all extraction space has been taken up, the interim .020 inch stainless Stage II archwires have only to derotate the first molars, with a buccal offset and toe-in, mesial to each molar tube.

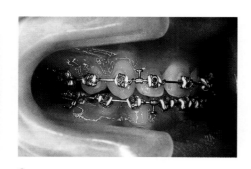
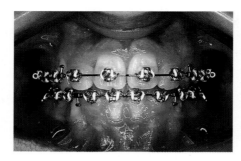
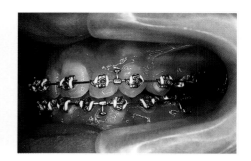

6

.0215 × .028 inch stainless archwires are fitted flat. In view of the Class III skeletal pattern, which may deteriorate with remaining growth, skeletal compensation is advisable in the anterior segments (mesial to the hooks). As described in Chapter 16, 8 degrees of retroclination can be obtained from a mandibular pretorqued archwire when fitted flat, without a bite sweep.

Proclination of the upper incisors can be achieved by fitting a 5 degree pretorqued maxillary arch inverted, or a suitably expanded 8 degree mandibular archwire. In this case, the latter is appropriate, with slight manual enhancement, producing approximately 10 degrees of proclination. In both archwires, the posterior segments (distal to the hooks) are returned to zero torque.

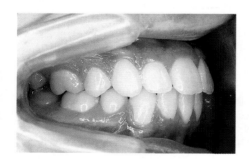
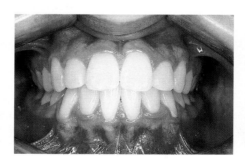
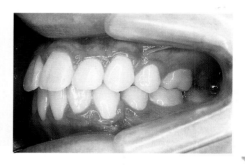

7

After 9 months in Stage III, all bracketed teeth have been individually torqued and tipped to the prescription described above. Class III intermaxillary elastics were confined to nights only use during Stage III. Note that the alignment of all four lateral incisor apices has been achieved without individualized archwire adjustment, and without inversion of the upper brackets. This is because the Side-Winder auxiliary closes each Tip-Edge slot into full approximation with the archwire, with no remaining free play.

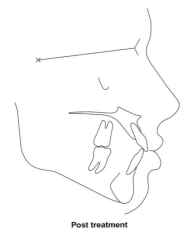

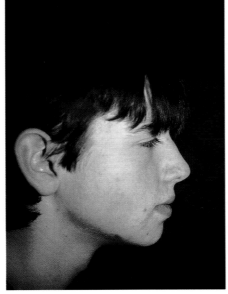

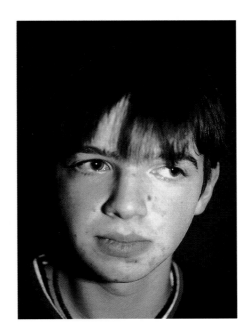

Post treatment

SKELETAL			TEETH		
SNA	°	85.0	Overjet	mm	2.5
SNB	°	82.0	Overbite	mm	2.0
ANB	°	2.5	UI/MxP	°	119.5
SN/MxP	°	10.0	LI/MnP	°	98.0
MxP/MnP	°	21.5	LI-APo	mm	5.5
LAFH/TAFH	%	56.5			

8
There is some improvement in lower face profile, despite worsening prognathism, due to the setting back of the lower anterior segment.

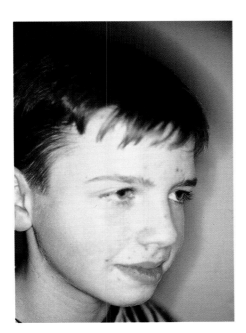

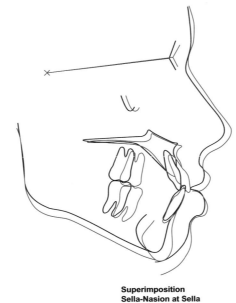

**Superimposition
Sella–Nasion at Sella**

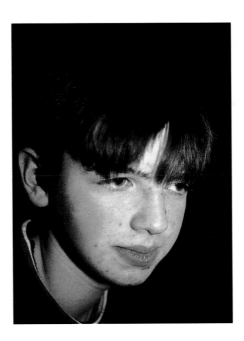

9
Taking account of mandibular growth, the lower incisors have been moved bodily lingually.

Treatment time = 1 year 8 months.
Routine adjustments = 10.
Archwires used = 6 (3 upper, 3 lower).
Retention = upper and lower Hawleys, nights only.

Stage III

Stage III

Objectives

1. Correction of torque and tip angles for each tooth individually.
2. Attainment of optimum facial profile compatible with stability.
3. Maintenance of Class I occlusion.
4. Final detailing.

In essence, Stage III produces the perfect finish, that 'film star smile' that we can confidently promise to our patients!

To conventional orthodontic thinking, it may be difficult to conceive that such a finish will be readily possible, either mechanically or physiologically, from an appliance that accommodates angles of torque and tip discrepancy that lie far outside the range of normal recovery with straight-wire brackets. Perhaps even more difficult to imagine is that such a recovery, in the hands of an experienced operator, is virtually maintenance free, accomplished by a single upper and lower rectangular archwire only, requiring no removal for adjustment.

Indeed, having exploited all the advantages of free tipping early in treatment, it is imperative that Tip-Edge should have a reliable uprighting and torquing mechanism, well beyond the capability of conventional brackets. Without this, it would be unable to match the finishing precision for which the straight-wire appliance has set the standard.

That the Tip-Edge appliance has this capability is due to the use of rectangular wire in an unexpected way, which is totally new in orthodontics.[1] For reasons which will be fully explained, it has the intrinsic capability to produce a more accurate finish than existing bracket systems, and arguably more so in the more challenging cases of greater initial severity. To aid understanding, this and the hitherto established method of torquing with rectangular archwires will be compared.

Conventional torquing

A conventional edgewise or straight-wire bracket has a fixed vertical bracket slot dimension, into which freeplay can only be introduced by using undersized archwires. As is well known, active torque is achieved by the use of an archwire of rectangular cross section, in which a third order torque deflection of the archwire will occur when inserted into the archwire slot. The torque force imparted will depend on the torque discrepancy between the archwire and the bracket, the elastic properties of the wire, and the degree to which the size of archwire fills the slot.

Although such a simple method may have served well over many generations, within its self-imposed limits, it is fundamentally flawed in one major area. Primarily, this is because the active component in torque production is the archwire itself, which is effectively acting as a spring. The rectangular wire is therefore required to provide active torque to those teeth requiring correction, while at the same time offering three-dimensional stability to the remainder. Combining these two conflicting functions in a single archwire is a physical impossibility. Many world respected researchers have identified and tried to address the problems of the unwanted reciprocals, whereby active torque imparted to a single unit, or quadrant, will inevitably impart unwanted secondary torque reactions in adjacent units, or groups of teeth, resulting in some 'round tripping'.[2-13]

Provided torque discrepancies are only minor, many orthodontists successfully ride through such problems, which are inherent in full rectangular archwire mechanics, rather than resorting to complicated segmental arch configurations, designed to eliminate such secondary reactions. However, there are other compromises in conventional torquing mechanics, which can less easily be ignored.

Returning, for a moment, to the conflicting requirements asked of a single rectangular wire in stabilizing some teeth while torquing others, there is a further dilemma concerning the ideal physical properties of the wire itself. For example, the relative flexibility of a nickel-titanium archwire may be preferable for progressive torquing with light forces. On the other hand, stainless steel might be the natural choice elsewhere in the arch for maintaining stability, particularly in the lateral and vertical dimensions, and robust enough to support intra- or intermaxillary traction concurrently.

Lastly, there is the question of archwire size. It is customary, in the majority of straight-wire techniques, not to exceed archwires of .019 × .025 inch, within a standard

.022 × .028 inch bracket slot. This is partly to limit the active forces fed to a tooth by too heavy an archwire, but also to allow ease of insertion and removal. As already stated in Chapter 1, this degree of tolerance will equate to nearly 10 degrees of 'torque slop' between archwire and bracket slot.[14] While evidently regarded as a physiological safety feature, it may nonetheless result in up to 10 degrees of undertreatment, unless compensated by individualized torque adjustment in the archwire, or a modified torque prescription in the bracket itself.[15]

How does Tip-Edge torque?

It is essential first to understand that a Tip-Edge bracket cannot be torqued by an active archwire in the conventional manner, even with a fully closed bracket slot. Examination of the design of the bracket will explain why (Fig. 14.1). The intact upper and lower finishing surfaces in each bracket are offset from one another, and are therefore never directly opposed. Insertion of an actively torqued rectangular archwire will therefore elevate one finishing surface and depress the other. In effect, the torquing effort in the archwire will have dispersed, by increasing the vertical dimension within the Tip-Edge slot. The net result will be a relapse of root uprighting in the mesio-distal direction, rather than any torque imparted to the root (Fig. 14.2). This is known as 'torque escape'.

Paradoxically, a new and entirely original method of torque delivery has been evolved from the selfsame bracket properties, by delivering torque simultaneously with tip correction. While the method might be thought cumbersome, since it utilizes auxiliary springs, it will be seen to be superior on many counts. Basically, it breaks new ground by relieving the rectangular wire of its double function: now the heavy base archwire becomes a passive platform, preserving three-dimensional rectangular control, while the Side-Winders provide the flexibility to torque and tip each bracket into conformity with the archwire. This is the first time in orthodontics that an auxiliary spring, acting in the second order plane of tip, has been used to generate third order

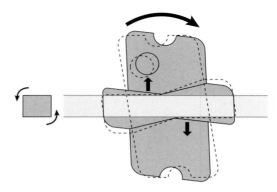

Fig. 14.2 'Torque escape', whereby an actively torqued rectangular archwire will reopen the vertical slot dimension, provoking second order root movement rather than third order torque.

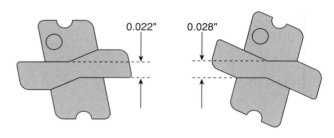

Fig. 14.3 During initial crown translation, the vertical archwire space will increase from .022 (A) up to a maximum .028 inches (B).

torque. Those with an interest in the underlying mathematics are referred to Parkhouse and Parkhouse.[16]

Clinically, what happens is this: during the first two stages of treatment, the bracketed teeth will have been free to tip, as previously described, thereby opening the vertical slot dimension from its nominal .022 inches, up to a possible .028 inches, depending upon the degree of translation (Fig. 14.3). It will be observed, in clinical use, that intrusion of anterior teeth during overbite reduction also tends to result in some mesial root movement, which adds to the bracket opening effect. Overall, even a small amount of mesial root or distal crown tipping will open up the vertical dimension a significant amount, due to the geometry of the Tip-Edge bracket.

At the onset of Stage III, therefore, a stainless .0215 × .028 inch archwire can be fitted without difficulty, since the vertical dimension available to the archwire, within each slot, will be comfortably in excess of the vertical dimension of the archwire itself. No torque will therefore be imparted at this point (Fig. 14.4A), and the archwire will not be deflected by any bracketed tooth. In fact, the only teeth subject to torque control from the outset will be the first molars, which wear buccal tubes.

Side-Winder springs are added to each tooth requiring correction (omitted from Fig. 14.4 in the interests of clarity).

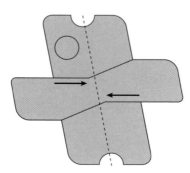

Fig. 14.1 The finishing surfaces of the bracket slot do not extend to the mid-point of the bracket.

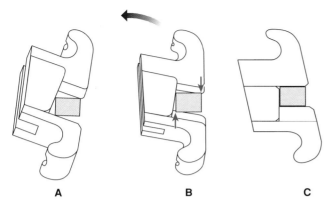

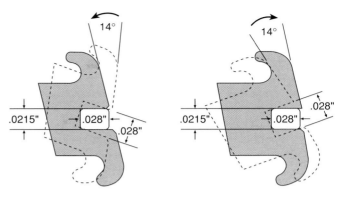

Fig. 14.4 Tip-Edge torquing. Viewed down the long axis of the archwire, a Side-Winder spring (omitted in the interests of clarity) is closing the vertical archwire space down again (i.e. Fig. 14.3B to Fig. 14.3A). (A) Initial engagement of rectangular wire. The vertical archwire space exceeds the vertical archwire dimension. There is no binding or archwire deflection. (B) The Side-Winder begins to close down the vertical archwire space, achieving an offset two-point contact with the archwire (small arrows). From here, torque (large arrow) and tip will be delivered concurrently. (C) Final tip and torque are achieved simultaneously when slot closes down completely onto the archwire.

Fig. 14.5 A Side-Winder spring (not shown) can recover 14 degrees of torque from either direction, without archwire deflection or archwire adjustment.

These are designed to 'think tip', since the coils are carried in the tip plane, so that the lever arm primarily generates tip. Each spring should therefore be selected to un-tip its crown towards the normal inclination, and in so doing, the vertical space in the bracket slot will automatically reduce, as the bracket begins to close down. Soon a point is reached when further progress in the tip plane becomes obstructed by the opposite corners of the rectangular archwire. A two-point contact is thus established within the bracket, as indicated by the small arrows (Fig. 14.4B). Because the Side-Winder is still active, these two points are attempting to close down still further, exerting light pressure against the archwire. Due to the fact that the two pressure points are offset in relation to the torque plane (one on the upper labial and the other on the lower lingual edge of the archwire), a secondary torquing couple is generated, which will induce palatal root torque in the direction of the heavy arrow (Fig. 14.4B). The archwire can thus be regarded as the meat within a progressively closing sandwich. As the torque begins to express, so further tip correction progresses, the two-point contact being continuously maintained under light pressure, until finally, when the bracket becomes fully closed down to the vertical dimension of the archwire, the upper and lower flat surfaces of the bracket slot will be in contact with the flat upper and lower surfaces of the archwire (Fig. 14.4C). Now, all torque and tip will have been fully expressed, with no residual 'torque slop'.

It is worth noting, in the sequence illustrated in Figure 14.4, that the rectangular archwire cross section remains undeflected throughout the entire torquing process. (Strictly, a small deflection of the archwire will be induced reciprocally, by the eccentric two point pressure contact. However, the force exerted by the light auxiliary spring is so small in relation to the torsional rigidity of the rectangular wire that this does not amount to clinical significance.) In practical terms we have, at last, an appliance that can torque teeth individually, without unwanted torque reactions to neighbouring teeth. Furthermore, it can torque either labially or lingually in the same manner, with a maximally open incisor bracket, at the beginning of Stage III, capable of accommodating 14 degrees of torque discrepancy in either direction (a total range of 28 degrees) without arch deflection (Fig. 14.5).

Both torque and tip actions are self-limited, according to the prescription in each bracket, by the approximation of upper and lower finishing surfaces to the archwire. However, a very small amount of overcorrection of tip (less than 1 degree) is permitted, since the .0125 inch vertical archwire dimension is fractionally smaller than the .022 inch archwire slot. When the Side-Winder has fully expressed, there will be zero torque discrepancy between bracket and archwire; the angle of torque finally adopted by the crown will therefore depend on the inclination of the rectangle of the archwire (as well as the prescription in the bracket base). Generally a zero torque angle in the archwire, defined as when the rectangular cross section lies flat and parallel to the mean occlusal plane, is appropriate to nearly all cases. This will yield the Rx-1 torque in base bracket prescription. However, we shall see later how this can be modified very simply, usually across anterior segments, to cater for certain skeletal situations. The necessity to carry inventories of different bracket prescriptions is thus avoided.

Points to note

- Each Side-Winder should always be orientated to un-tip the tooth, irrespective of which direction torque is required. The passive set of the rectangle in the archwire provides the benchmark to which the tooth will be torqued.

- Once a two point contact is achieved (Fig. 14.4B), tip and torque delivery are unalterably related, according to the geometry of the bracket–archwire interface, the root apex describing a slightly curved path into its predetermined finished position.[16]
- Completion of torque and tip occurs simultaneously, for each tooth.
- If a bracket is prevented from expressing its torque fully (either by premature removal of the spring, or by an unattainable torque target), there will be a corresponding shortfall in tip correction. The same is true vice versa: inadequate tip correction will prevent full torque correction.
- A Side-Winder needs to work slightly harder to produce a combination of tip and torque than when producing tip alone.[16]
- Force values decline progressively as the spring unwinds, from a possible maximum of 60 grams down to 20 grams, at the apex.[16]
- Force values can be restored, if desired, by 'hyperactivating' the spring (described in Chapter 18) during treatment.
- Hyperactivation is appropriate on incisors when obtaining the final torque prescription.
- It may be helpful to continue with Side-Winder springs at full activation, even after self-limiting, particularly on lower incisors, to boost anchorage by maintaining bodily control.
- Because zero tolerance remains between bracket slot and rectangular archwire when each bracket has expressed and self-limited, inverted brackets are never required on palatally displaced upper lateral incisors. Reversing the torque by 16 degrees in this way is likely to impact the root against the labial plate. Because the Side-Winder will then be prevented from closing the bracket down further, a shortfall of tip correction will result.
- High torque brackets may be contraindicated for similar reasons. It is easier to vary the torque set in the archwire, to compensate skeletal variations (as described in Chapter 15).
- It is a mistake to use an archwire of less than .0215 × .028 inch. Narrowing the width of the torquing platform reduces the effectiveness of the spring and retards progress. A thinner archwire also becomes more liable to distortion by the spring.

In summary

Use of rectangular wire as a passive benchmark, to which each bracket will be individually adapted, is a unique innovation. Is there any parallel with straight-wire practice? In fact, as will be seen, there is.

With edgewise or straight-wire bracket systems, it has long been recognized that even undersized rectangular archwires will generate some degree of torque control, so long as the archwires are active vertically during levelling. In such a situation, the flat upper and lower archwire surfaces will be working against opposite corners of the rectangular bracket slot, imparting some measure of torque control. Before the advent of nickel-titanium wires, it was accepted practice to engage rectangular stainless archwires in progressively larger sections, obtaining greater torque definition in the process (also with increasing forces). If it were possible to fill the slot completely, the torque prescription would be fully realized. In principle, therefore, the archwires are increased in size to fill the conventional bracket slot.

Tip-Edge approaches the same problem from a reverse perspective. Instead of increasing archwire thickness to fill the bracket, a Tip-Edge bracket shrinks its vertical dimension (under pressure from an auxiliary spring) to fit a full sized archwire, conforming to it precisely in all three dimensions.

Anchorage considerations

While the first two stages of treatment progress with dramatically small demands on anchorage, due to the fact that the teeth are permitted to tip, it should not be assumed that root uprighting is without its demands on anchorage. Indeed, these must be predicted and allowed for. For this reason, a cephalometric radiograph should always be taken on entry to Stage III, and compared with the pretreatment radiograph and against final treatment objectives.

Because all teeth in each arch will be in contact, anchorage will no longer affect groups of teeth, but each arch as a whole, sometimes known as 'contiguous anchorage'. Therefore, anchorage sequelae may influence the interarch relationship, which needs to be maintained in correction throughout the root uprighting phase, as well as influencing the facial profile.

With understanding and experience, it is possible to predict the likely direction and extent of anchorage shift, according to the direction and degree of root movement required in each arch, although there is individual variation, not least the underlying growth pattern, which fundamentally affects the interarch relationship. Nevertheless, in Class II cases, the normal expectation is for both arches to become more procumbent, particularly the maxillary arch.

This can be gauged from Figure 14.6, in which the arrows denote the required root corrections. In this first premolar extraction example, the lower arch is fairly straightforward, in that the reciprocal forces of the canine and second premolar partly cancel one another out, as the roots are being moved in opposite directions. Since the canine is the larger rooted tooth, however, there may still be an overall tendency towards mesial migration, particularly if it requires a greater angle of tip correction. The same applies to the upper arch, to which must be added the reciprocal of any incisor root torque, which will tend to advance the upper incisors, and so increase arch procumbence. A balance between the arches must therefore be struck, to preserve a correct interarch

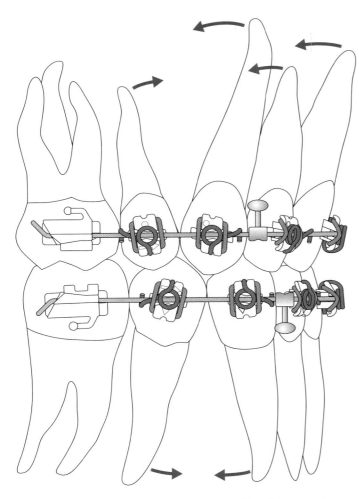

Fig. 14.6 Anchorage implications in a Class II four first premolar extraction case: the arrows indicate the various root movements, each of which affects anchorage.

maintain the same objective. In practice, headgear is required very seldom in Tip-Edge, but it may occasionally be a useful adjunct to boost anchorage during Stage III, where a Class II case threatens to become too procumbent if intermaxillary traction is continued.

From the foregoing it follows that, in Class II cases powered by intermaxillary elastics, Stage III should be approached from a somewhat retrusive position, in order to allow for the anchorage shift during root uprighting (Fig. 14.7), without calling for additional anchorage support from elsewhere. Anchorage requirements in other malocclusion types are generally less.

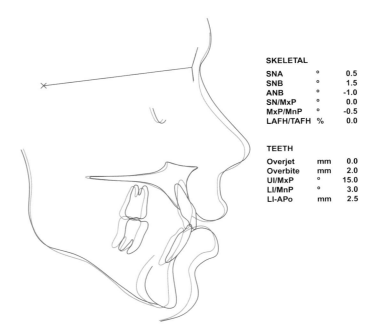

SKELETAL		
SNA	°	0.5
SNB	°	1.5
ANB	°	-1.0
SN/MxP	°	0.0
MxP/MnP	°	-0.5
LAFH/TAFH	%	0.0

TEETH		
Overjet	mm	0.0
Overbite	mm	2.0
UI/MxP	°	15.0
LI/MnP	°	3.0
LI-APo	mm	2.5

Fig. 14.7 Stage III anchorage considerations: over 7 months in Stage III in a four first premolar extraction case. The maxillary incisors have torqued 15 degrees, concurrent with distal root uprighting of all four canines, as depicted in Figure 14.6. Some forward projection of the dentition has taken place due to a combination of root corrections, mandibular growth and Class II intermaxillary elastics, worn at nights to maintain the interarch relationship.

relationship. In a case treated by means of intermaxillary elastics, these should be worn sufficiently to hold upper and lower incisors in contact; frequently this will involve elastics at night times only. Similarly a headgear patient will need to wear the headgear as many nights a week as it takes to

REFERENCES

1. Parkhouse RC. Rectangular wire and third order torque: a new perspective. American Journal of Orthodontics 1998; 113: 421–430.

2. Burstone CJ, Koenig HA. Force systems from an ideal arch. American Journal of Orthodontics 1974; 65: 270–289.

3. Burstone CJ. Rationale of the segmented arch. American Journal of Orthodontics 1962; 48: 805–822.

4. Burstone CJ. The mechanics of the segmented arch techniques. Angle Orthodontist 1996; 36: 99–120.

5. Creekmore TD. jco/interviews Dr Thomas D Creekmore on torque. Journal of Clinical Orthodontics 1979; 13: 305–310.

6. Demange C. Equilibrium situations in bend force systems. American Journal of Orthodontic and Dentofacial Orthopedics 1990; 98: 333–339.

7. Isaacson RJ, Lindauer SJ, Rubenstein LK. Moments with the edgewise appliance: incisor torque control. American Journal of Orthodontic Dentofacial Orthopedics 1993; 103: 428–438.

8. Isaacson RJ. Creative arch wires and clinical conclusion. Seminars in Orthodontics 1995; 1: 55–56.

9. Isaacson RJ, Rebellato J. Two-Couple orthodontic appliance systems: torquing arches. Seminars in Orthodontics 1995; 1: 31–36.

10. Rauch ED. Torque and its application to orthodontics. American Journal of Orthodontics 1959; 45: 817–830.

11. Schrody DW. A mechanical evaluation of buccal segment reaction to edgewise torque. Angle Orthodontist 1974; 44: 120–126.

12. Smith RJ, Burstone CJ. Mechanics of tooth movement. American Journal of Orthodontics 1984; 85: 294–307.

13. Yoshikawa DK. Biomechanical principles of tooth movement. Dental Clinics of North America 1981; 25: 19–26.

14. McLaughlin RP, Bennett JC, Trevisi HJ. Systemized orthodontic treatment mechanics. Edinburgh: Mosby; 2001.

15. Creekmore TD, Kunik RL. Straight wire: the next generation. American Journal of Orthodontics 1993; 194: 8–20.

16. Parkhouse RC, Parkhouse PS. American Journal of Orthodontics and Dentofacial Orthopedics 2001; 119: 632–639.

CASE 9

A high mandibular angle Class II division 1 malocclusion with bimaxillary protrusion and crowding

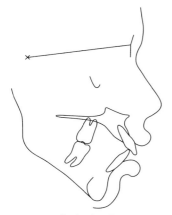

Pre-treatment

SKELETAL			TEETH		
SNA	°	78.5	Overjet	mm	5.5
SNB	°	74.0	Overbite	mm	2.0
ANB	°	4.5	UI/MxP	°	119.5
SN/MxP	°	7.0	LI/MnP	°	98.0
MxP/MnP	°	38.5	LI-APo	mm	8.5
LAFH/TAFH	%	54.0			

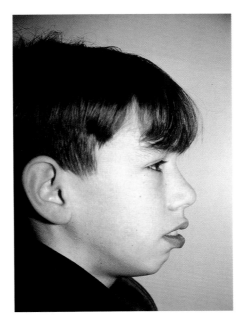

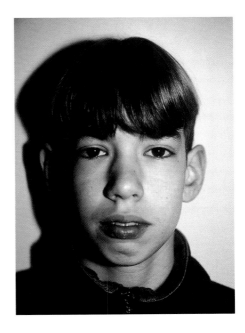

1

Extraoral anchorage is rarely required with Tip-Edge, and this is the only case illustrated in which headgear is worn.

At 13 years 9 months, there is a skeletal Class II base with a high maxillary–mandibular planes angle (38.5 degrees). The lower incisors are proclined to 8.5 mm ahead of the A–Po line with incompetent lips. With an already high mandibular angle, further clockwise rotation must be avoided. Intrusive anchorage forces are therefore used, instead of anchor bends and intermaxillary elastics, which might provoke unwanted extrusion of molars in a 'high angle' case.

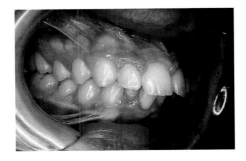

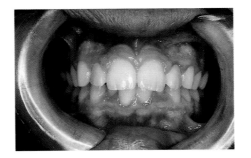

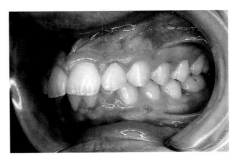

2

In addition to 5.5 mm of overjet, the lower lateral incisors are crowded lingually. Unusually, in such a skeletal pattern, the overbite is increased and complete.

Four first premolar extractions are indicated, since the lower incisors are +8.5 mm to A–Po and the overjet needs reducing to a corrected lower incisor position.

Lower arch anchorage will be intramandibular, but upper arch anchorage will be derived from combination headgear applied to the upper first molars by means of a Kloehn bow, a high pull component (approximately 500 grams) exceeding the cervical component, to produce a resultant intrusive and distal anchorage force vector.

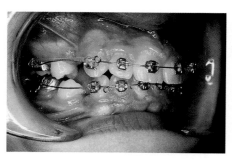
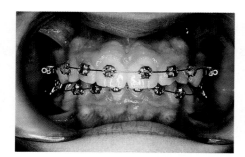
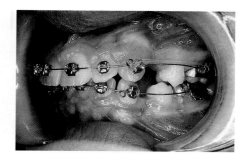

3

.016 inch Stage I stainless archwires are used, but without lower anchorage bends. Instead of Class II elastics, upper intra-arch E-7 elastomerics begin overjet reduction. The bite opening bends mesial to the upper first molars are not strictly anchor bends, since the headgear to the molars provides the anchorage, ensuring that these will neither shift mesially nor extrude. Rather, the bite opening bends distribute some of the intrusive effect of the headgear to the anterior segment, ensuring that the incisors intrude as the overjet reduces. This is a highly effective treatment for 'gummy smile'.

   With Tip-Edge, headgear wear during sleep only, 8 hours per night, will be found to be adequate.

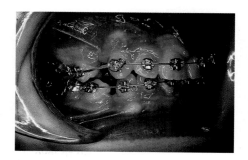
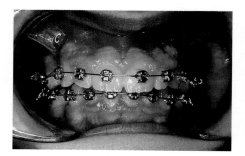
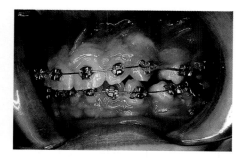

4

Without Class II elastics and anchorage bends, overbite reduction is slower, produced by gentle arch levelling in the mandible, whereas after 5 months, overjet reduction and upper incisor intrusion are proceeding apace. The premolars are bonded for alignment to the rectangular tubes. In retrospect, the lower premolars might have been bonded from the outset, with use of rectangular tubes throughout, since levelling of this lower arch does not require elastics or anchor bends.

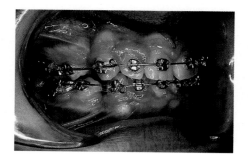
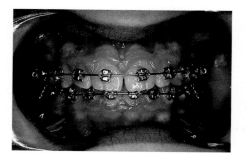
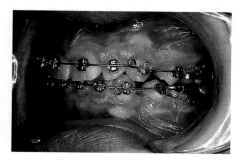

5

One visit later, .020 inch stainless archwires are fitted with intramaxillary traction E-5 elastomerics for space closure. Since the lower incisors were initially proclined, this is a 'retractive Stage II', without Side-Winder brakes, and nightly headgear is continued.

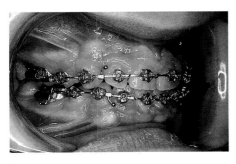
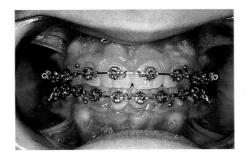
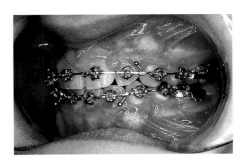

6

Nine months into treatment, .0215 × .028 inch stainless Stage III archwires are fitted with sweeps to retain the reduced overbite. Pretorqued archwires will enable zero torque to be maintained in the presence of bite sweeps. Headgear continues to support anchorage during root torquing and uprighting. 50 grams Class III intermaxillary elastics, worn at nights, redistribute some of the headgear anchorage to the mandible, preventing unwanted labial movement of the lower arch.

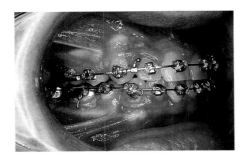
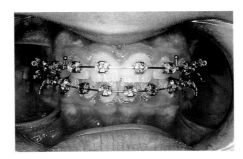
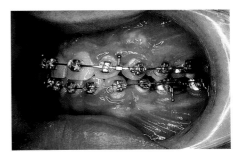

7

Late in Stage III, the lower first molars show some distal crown tip. The lower second molars are therefore banded to level the first molars with a .020 inch stainless archwire, converting the lower first molar tubes to brackets.

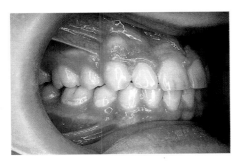
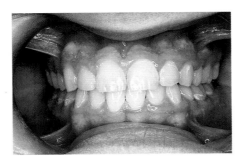
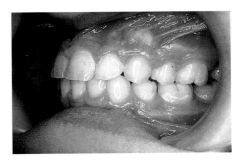

8

Co-operation with headgear has been excellent, producing a slight overcorrection of the interarch relationship.

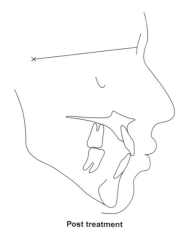

Post treatment

SKELETAL			TEETH		
SNA	°	76.5	Overjet	mm	2.5
SNB	°	76.0	Overbite	mm	1.0
ANB	°	0.5	UI/MxP	°	112.5
SN/MxP	°	9.5	LI/MnP	°	86.0
MxP/MnP	°	33.5	LI-APo	mm	5.0
LAFH/TAFH	%	55.0			

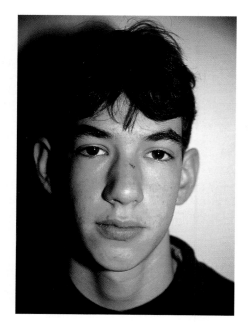

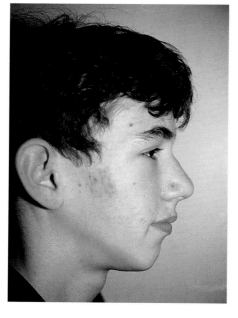

9
There is a noticeably better lip seal and this case appears less Class II skeletally.

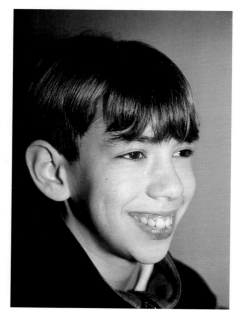

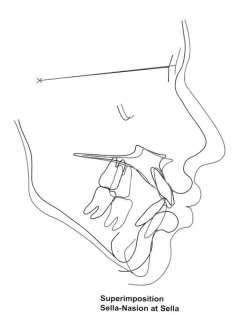

Superimposition
Sella-Nasion at Sella

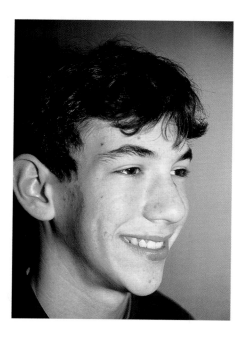

10
The gummy smile has improved dramatically and the headgear has had some orthopaedic effect. Forward growth of the maxilla has been restricted, and arguably the vertical development of the posterior maxilla has been restrained also. This in turn appears to have allowed a small autorotation of the mandible. Not only has clockwise rotation of the growing mandible been prevented, but also a small counter-clockwise rotation has occurred.

Treatment time = 1 year 8 months.
Routine adjustments = 14.
Archwires used = 7 (3 upper, 4 lower).
Retention = upper and lower Hawleys, nights only.

Stage III archwires

Stage III archwires

At the setting up visit for Stage III, the patient may be only halfway through treatment, in terms of time taken. The orthodontist will be thinking up to 9 months ahead, since he will effectively be programming the final result. Care and attention at this point will be amply rewarded; once correctly set up, the third stage will progress and self-limit automatically, with a minimum of supervision and adjustment.

The various steps will be described in turn as a clinical sequence, in this and the two following chapters, beginning with tailoring the archwires to shape and size, adjusting the passive torque setting subsequently, then fitting and removing the archwires.

Choice of archwires

Only one size of rectangular wire is ever used in Stage III. This is .0215 × .028 inch 'Shiny Bright' stainless (the lateral dimension is actually .027 inch, to facilitate insertion in the molar tubes). However, such archwires come in two formats: plain or pretorqued. The choice between these will be described later, and is summarized at the end of the next chapter. Basically, pretorqued will be indicated when bite sweeps are used, cancelling out the incisor proclination, or labial crown torque, that would otherwise result from the sweeps. These arches are also used for different reasons in Class III cases, where an atypical torque prescription may be appropriate to the anterior segments.

Arch width

The Standard (straight leg) arch shape should be used as the starting point. This will almost invariably be too narrow for the patient. However, it is easier to expand a rectangular arch, simply by placing it on a flat surface and widening the legs, rather than trying to contract one, which risks altering the torque. Initial expansion should be about 2 mm per side, across the molars (Fig. 15.1) in each arch. If gauged from the initial models, allowance should be made for any molar width corrections in the treatment design.

Identifying the 'landmarks'

The archwire can be rough cut for length against the models, so that it can be tried in comfortably. Holding the centreline

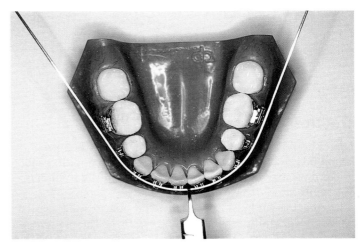

Fig. 15.1 Before 'customizing', each archwire should be expanded to approximately 2 mm each side, across the first molars.

marking precisely at the midline, the arch ends should now be cut accurately, leaving 3 mm of wire protruding from the distal of each molar tube. With an arch marking crayon, the contacts between first molars and premolars should be identified on the archwire for the placement of toe-ins, and the contact between canines and lateral incisors should be marked for the addition of traction hooks (Fig. 15.2).

Archform

Approximately 5 degrees of lingual toe-in should be placed opposite the mesial molar contacts. This ensures that the archwire enters the preangulated molar tubes at an equivalent angle to straight-wire archform. It will also restore archwire width across the molars to its desired measurement, while maintaining between 1 and 2 mm of expansion across the premolars, yet avoiding any increase in intercanine width. (This archform has been found to work well for UK patients, who generally have relatively narrow arches. However, those wishing to use the 'horseshoe shaped' straight-wire configuration may prefer to introduce some buccal segment curvature. For ease of fit, this should be preceded by a similar curvature to the .020 inch Stage II archwire at its final adjustment.)

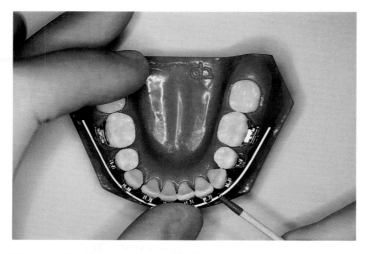

Fig. 15.2 Identifying the landmarks for hooks and toe-ins.

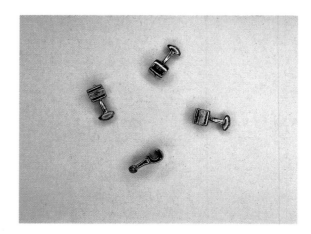

Fig. 15.3 T-shaped crimpable hooks.

Traction hooks

These should be crimped on to the wire midway between lateral incisor and canine brackets. Siting them any closer to the canines may interfere with the arms of the Side-Winders. The hooks should always point gingivally.

Such hooks are T-shaped, and therefore able to accept elastics or elastomerics from either direction (Fig. 15.3). They are seated from the buccal and need to be crimped tightly, using a special plier (Fig. 15.4). An internal tungsten coating prevents slippage along the wire. While the design of such hooks enables them to be crimped on in the mouth, this is not recommended. As will be seen later, the hooks act as useful 'markers' for the points at which torque is checked and adjusted. Squeezing them on afterwards may therefore distort the torque setting.

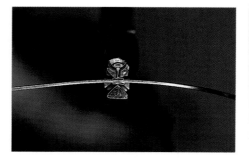

Fig. 15.4 Lingual view of hook crimped with special plier.

Preparation of arch ends

This is vital, to enable easy insertion and removal. It is essential to cinch the arch ends gingivally during Stage III in all cases, as the reciprocal action of the auxiliary springs, in uprighting the roots, will otherwise separate the crowns, and introduce unwanted spacing.

The 3 mm of wire projecting distal to the first molar tubes will therefore need thinning and thorough annealing. A full thickness of wire is not necessary in a cinch back, and merely makes subsequent removal needlessly difficult. The distal ends can therefore be ground out from the lingual to about half the original width (Fig. 15.5). They are ground out from the lingual because, when feeding the wire into a buccal tube, it is invariably the lingual corner of the cut end that catches in the tube.

As for annealing, this can be done with a flame, taking care not to extend the softened section too far mesially. Alternatively, the heat trapped in the distal section, generated by a high revving grinding wheel, can do the same.

Maxillary and mandibular arches should now be correlated (Fig. 15.6). They are now prepared, except for the torque and bite sweep.

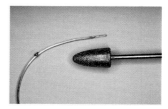

Fig. 15.5 The protruding distal archwire ends are thinned and annealed.

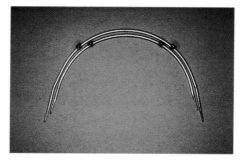

Fig. 15.6 Correlated Stage III archwires.

Stage III: setting the torques

Stage III: setting the torque

How to 'read' the torque

The torque set in any part of an archwire can easily be visualized by holding the prepared archwire within the beaks of a torquing plier, at the point at which torque is to be assessed. Testing anterior torque at the midline, with the archwire held 'back to front' (legs towards the plier handles), zero torque will be confirmed when the distal ends of the archwire lie midway between the handles. This simply demonstrates that the angle of the rectangle, at the point held, is aligned parallel to the occlusal plane. Figure 16.1 illustrates zero anterior torque, as tested at the midline.

In essence, each rectangular archwire in Tip-Edge has three torque segments: the incisor segment and both buccal segments. The hooks demarcate these three zones.

It is just as easy to read the torque in the buccal segments, simply by holding one leg at its distal end. Figure 16.2 demonstrates zero torque at the distal end being held, since the opposite distal end lies midway between the plier handles. Zero torque in the buccal segments is almost invariably desirable, rare exceptions being major arch width discrepancies or skeletal asymmetries.

Torque in reduced overbite cases

In cases in which the initial overbite was reduced, or open, no vertical bite sweeps will be required. Plain, flat, untorqued

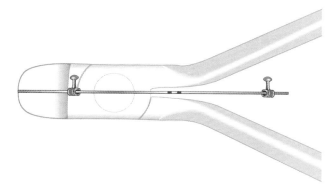

Fig. 16.2 The same archwire held at the distal: the opposite distal end lies midway between the handles, denoting zero torque at the buccal segment held.

archwires can therefore be fitted, without torque adjustment. These will effectively be set at 'zero torque' throughout, as supplied, thus delivering the Rx-1 torque in base bracket prescription to each bracketed tooth individually. An exception may be in skeletal Class III cases, for which non-standard angulations may be preferred across the incisor segments, as will be described later in this chapter.

Using a mid-crown bonding position, flat archwires will produce a marginal increase in overbite, hence a small overcorrection of a reduced overbite.

Torque in increased overbite cases

A zero torque archwire setting throughout will still be the aim. However, where overbite reduction has been required in Stage I (and therefore maintained with bite sweeps throughout Stage II), it follows that similar vertical bite sweeps will be needed to maintain the reduced overbite during the third stage also. This introduces complications, since sweeping a vertical curvature along the buccal segments of any rectangular wire will automatically alter the torque setting at the front, producing unwanted incisor proclination. This is shown in a lower archwire, zero torqued when flat (Fig. 16.3A) and after placement of a vertical bite sweep (Fig. 16.3B). It will be seen (Fig. 16.3B) that the distal archwire ends no longer bisect the plier handles, but are now

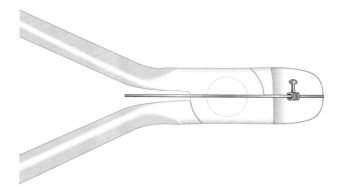

Fig. 16.1 A 'zero torque' archwire, held at the midline: the archwire ends distal to the first molars lie midway between the handles, denoting zero torque at the front.

137

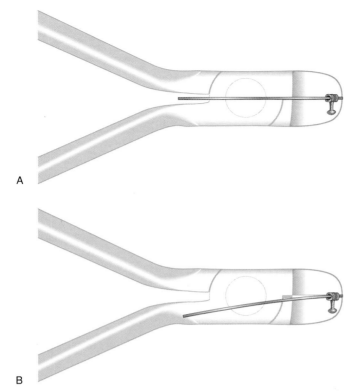

A

B

Fig. 16.3 (A) A zero torque lower archwire only remains zero torque when flat. (B) Placing a vertical bite sweep (reverse curve of Spee) automatically produces labial crown torque at the front (the distal arch ends no longer lie midway between the handles).

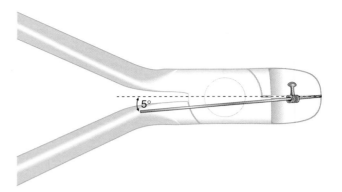

Fig. 16.4 A pretorqued maxillary archwire contains 5 degrees of lingual crown torque throughout.

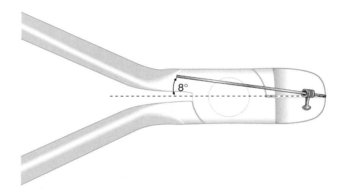

Fig. 16.5 A pretorqued mandibular archwire contains 8 degrees of lingual crown torque throughout.

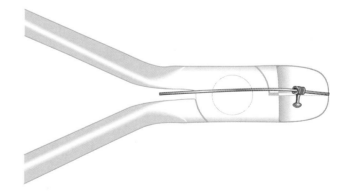

Fig. 16.6 When a vertical bite sweep is placed (to retain a previously reduced overbite), the in-built lingual crown torque cancels out the labial crown torque produced by the sweep. The distal ends lie midway between the handles.

below them, denoting labial crown torque, which will cause proclination of the lower incisors.

What is therefore required is some lingual crown torque in the anterior segment, to counteract the labial crown torque produced by the bite sweep, thereby restoring zero torque to the lower incisors. Zero torque should also be set along the buccal segments. In former times, this combination required intricate torque manipulations. Fortunately, none of this is any longer necessary, since the advent of pretorqued archwires.

Pretorqued archwires

These are identical dimensionally to the plain rectangular archwires already illustrated, but come with 5 degrees of lingual crown torque in the maxillary (Fig. 16.4) and 8 degrees of lingual crown torque in the mandibular arch (Fig. 16.5). Used in a case with an initially increased overbite, the purpose of the inbuilt retroclination will be to cancel out the proclination produced by the bite sweep (Fig. 16.6). Because of the continuity of the wire, the pretorque in each archwire extends overall, including the buccal segments (Fig. 16.7), from which it must later be removed. However, this avoids the necessity for the orthodontist to stock an

inventory of different sizes; tailoring each arch and placing the hooks appropriately allows one size to be adapted to all.

Pretorqued archwires are identified by their centreline markings, which appear on the upper surfaces only. The maxillary archwire therefore carries its single mark on the gingival surface, while the mandibular has double markings, both on the occlusal surface (Fig. 16.8). By this means, both upper and lower centreline markings will be visible to the operator when the archwires are in the mouth (Fig. 16.9), thereby avoiding accidental misfitting of an archwire upside down, which would, of course, reverse the torque.

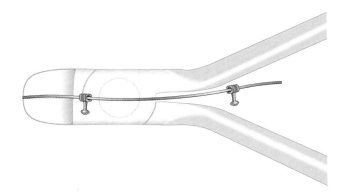

Fig. 16.7 Lingual crown pretorque extends down the buccal segments where it will need to be returned to zero torque as shown in Figure 16.12.

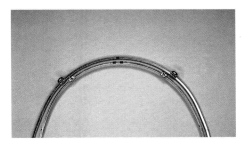

Fig. 16.8 Centreline markings on pretorqued archwires are on the upper surfaces only, to safeguard against accidental inversion. Fitting either archwire upside down would reverse the torque.

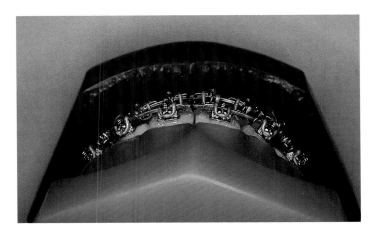

Fig. 16.9 Other than some Class III cases (see text), upper and lower centreline markings on pretorqued archwires should be visible to the operator, confirming that neither archwire is fitted upside down.

Wiping the sweep, checking the torque

The sweep comes first. The archwire should be held in a torquing plier, immediately mesial to the hook, and a vertical bite sweep curvature stroked into the buccal segment with thumb and finger, working distally, to produce a reverse curve of Spee in the lower arch and a 'rocking horse' curve in the upper. As with the Stage II bite sweep, most of the curvature should be along the canine and premolar regions, not extending into the molar tubes. In practice, the effect of the sharp distal end against the thumb or finger prevents this naturally! The same action should be repeated on the opposite side, to create a matching sweep. The amount of archwire intrusion at the front should normally amount to 1–2 mm (Fig. 16.10).

Now to check the torque. Firstly, check the incisor segment, by holding the wire at the midline, to see if there is zero torque (Fig. 16.6). Small torque adjustments can be made by gently deflecting the tails of the archwire vertically with thumb and finger, while holding the centreline steady in a plier (Fig. 16.11). (Distal ends up, in the maxillary arch, will increase torque and vice versa. In the mandibular arch, it is the opposite.)

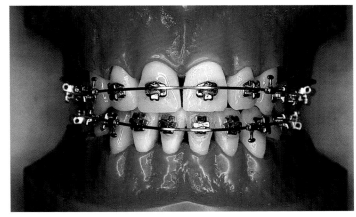

Fig. 16.10 A small amount of anterior archwire intrusion is all that is necessary to retain a previously deep bite throughout Stage III.

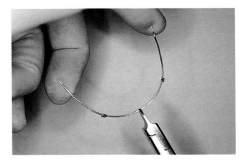

Fig. 16.11 A small amount of palatal root torque can be added to the upper incisor segment by elevating the tails of the archwire.

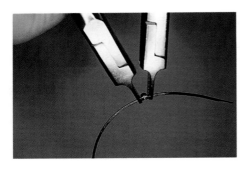

Fig. 16.12 Knocking out any residual pretorque in the buccal segment. The hooks are the landmarks: a small twist between the pliers at the hook restores the buccal segment to zero torque.

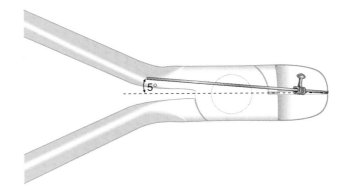

Fig. 16.13 Inverting a pretorqued upper archwire and fitting it flat will result in 5 degrees of incisor proclination, as may be appropriate to a Class III case.

Generally, the normal degree of bite sweep in the upper will automatically produce zero torque at the front, although in Class II division 2 cases it may be expedient to add a little more sweep, which will result in 2 or 3 degrees of extra torque, giving some overcorrection of interincisal angle (as in Cases 5 and 6). In the lower, however, a normal amount of bite sweep may not quite cancel out the pretorque retroclination, and a degree or two of residual labial root torque, to which this equates, may be beneficial to lower incisor stability in Class II cases.

Lastly, any pretorque remaining in the buccal segments needs to be returned to zero torque. This is a simple adjustment, on each side, performed by placing torquing pliers either side of the hook, and in contact with it. A small twist between the pliers, along the long axis of the wire, can readily produce zero torque of the buccal segment (Fig. 16.12). The same applies to the opposite side.

Often, however, it will be found that any adjustment required to achieve zero buccal segment torque will be small, or even unnecessary. This is because, when making the bite sweep, the action of sweeping around the curved section immediately distal to the hooks tends in itself to reduce the pretorque in the distal section towards zero.

Finally, it is as well to re-check the bite sweep, in case this has been disturbed during the torque adjustment.

Class III cases

Many straight-wire bracket manufacturers provide alternative anterior torque prescriptions to cater for Class III cases. Although a Tip-Edge Rx-3 bracket does exist, it is far easier to vary the torque setting in the anterior segment of the archwire than to carry different sets of brackets. This is particularly relevant to Class III cases. Here it may be desirable to compensate a prognathic mandible by treating the lower incisors to a retroclined position, while some proclination of the upper incisors may also need to be incorporated, to sustain a positive overjet. Such variations can easily be accommodated by using pretorqued archwires, but in a different way.

Typically, Class III malocclusions feature a reduction in overbite, for which bite sweeps will be inappropriate. By using the archwires unswept, therefore, the pretorque can be maintained across the anterior segments, to produce a non-standard incisor angulation.

In the mandibular arch, this is easy. The lower pretorqued archwire contains 8 degrees of lingual crown torque throughout. Fitted without a bite sweep, this will cause the Side-Winders to produce 8 degrees of retroclination (Fig. 16.5). The only torque adjustment required will be to produce zero torque in the buccal segments, achieved by means of the two pairs of torquing pliers, either side of the hooks, as described earlier (Fig. 16.12).

The maxillary arch is no less easy, but requires some 'inverted thinking'. This is because the pretorque set in the archwire is lingual crown torque, and retroclination is not what the upper incisors want in a Class III case. To reverse the torque, it is only necessary to flip the archwire upside down. By this means, 5 degrees of retroclination becomes 5 degrees of proclination (Fig. 16.13). An unswept upper pretorqued archwire, fitted upside down, is therefore generally suitable for the maxillary arch in Class III cases. This is therefore the sole instance, in Stage III, when a centreline marking will not be visible to the operator on insertion.

Severe skeletal Class II cases

Having described anterior modification in archwire torque prescription to accommodate a Class III skeletal pattern, the question whether similar consideration should be given to the severe skeletal Class II patient might be asked. In such cases it may be impossible to achieve correct torque values on upper incisors due to the proximity of the palatal cortex. Equally, some proclination of the lower incisors may be beneficial to help camouflage a retrognathic mandible, which could easily be achieved by placing a bite sweep in an uncompensated zero torque archwire.

However, in the author's experience it has seldom proved necessary to modify the archwires since, in the hierarchy of forces with Tip-Edge, the effect of intermaxillary elastics (which may well be required full time through Stage III in adverse growth patterns) will overwhelm the activity of the Side-Winders. In effect, the springs will produce as much torque as they are enabled, whereupon root movement will cease if an obstruction is encountered.

Theoretically, a slight shortfall in tip correction will result whenever torque is not fully expressed against the archwire, but in practice this is scarcely noticed. Neither has root resorption been observed during Stage III in such cases. Because the torquing action of Side-Winder auxiliaries is so gentle, compared with archwire torquing in conventional brackets, the orthodontist need never fear the spectre of roots penetrating cortical bone as a result of a minor conflict in torque prescription.

Summary of pretorqued versus plain archwires

- For reduced overbite and anterior open bite cases, choose plain arches, fitted flat.

- In cases that have required overbite reduction, vertical bite sweeps will be needed to maintain the reduced overbite. Therefore, pretorqued archwires will be necessary to cancel out the incisor proclination resulting from the bite sweeps.

- In Class III cases, with normal or reduced overbites, pretorqued arches can be used flat, without a sweep. However, the upper archwire should be inverted. Five degrees of proclination and 8 degrees of retroclination will then be given to the upper and lower incisors respectively.

Stage III: fitting the archwires

Stage III: fitting the archwires

There should be no difficulty in fitting the rectangular wires, so long as levelling and alignment has been satisfactorily maintained during the second stage. Resistance when attempting to enter the molar tubes is almost invariably due to failure to derotate the molars at the last Stage II adjustment.

Quite contrary to what might be expected with conventional brackets, all bracketed teeth should accept the .0215 × .028 inch archwire readily, since their vertical archwire space will be increased beyond the vertical dimension of the wire. Indeed, at the fit visit, none of the bracketed teeth will 'know' that they are engaged with rectangular wire, for there will be no binding. No torque effect will be imparted either, until the Side-Winders set to work, because the archwire itself is passive in the brackets.

However, this is not so with the first molars, which are subject to accurate torque control from the moment the archwire is fitted.

Testing molar torque

Before fitting the archwire, it is important to assess whether there is any torque discrepancy between the archwire and the buccal tubes, and any active torque thus found should be recorded in the patient's notes. Just as with any edgewise-based appliance, the test is to insert the distal end of the archwire into the buccal tube on one side only, keeping clear of the brackets, and then observing the height of the free distal end on the opposite side, relative to its buccal tube (Fig. 17.1). Any height discrepancy at this point will denote the direction and extent of the torque discrepancy in the molar engaged. The same test should then be applied to the opposite first molar.

Should any torque discrepancy be apparent, this does not necessarily imply a fault requiring rectification. The temptation to adjust the buccal segment torque away from zero, to make it passive in the tube, should generally be resisted. More often than not, the archwire may be telling the orthodontist something about the molars. Have the mandibular molars inclined lingually, for instance? If so, a zero torque setting in the archwire will upright them. Figure 17.2 shows the engagement of an upper second molar in a

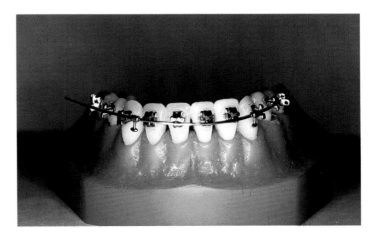

Fig. 17.1 Testing for torque discrepancy in a molar tube.

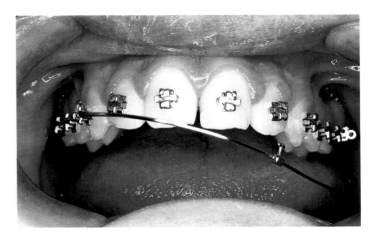

Fig. 17.2 A major torque discrepancy is revealed between this zero torque archwire and the upper second molar tube (see text).

first molar extraction case, in which the palatal cusp has dropped; again, this will be corrected automatically during the stage, without need for archwire adjustment. Sometimes when fitting the archwires, if there is a considerable torque discrepancy, a small flexion of the archwire about its long axis may be necessary to enable it to slide freely into its buccal tube.

The question may be asked as to whether such a solid rectangular wire, imparting torque to a molar, is too heavy to be safe, either to the molar or to adjacent teeth. The unexpected answer is that, because the bracket slots are opened up vertically, and therefore not 'grabbing' the archwire at any point, the interbracket span is effectively from one first molar all the way round to the other, and the bracketed teeth themselves remain unaffected.

Cinch backs

As previously explained, all cases require cinch backs, at the distal arch ends, to prevent unwanted spaces opening up due to the action of the Side-Winders. However, the management of these cinch backs is critical to preventing tight contacts, which will halt progress and may induce rotations. In this, it should be remembered that crowns require additional arch length as they upright mesio-distally, particularly canines and premolars. This should be allowed for in the cinch back. It is strongly recommended that the cinch backs should be placed and tested *before* fitting the springs and modules. This makes it easy to ascertain how much free space will be admitted.

A tiny amount of space (a 0.5–1 mm) somewhere in each arch is good. If this is already present, the annealed arch ends should be turned gingivally at the point of exit from the tube. This is best done with a light wire plier, held open. With the square beak resting gingival to the tube and the round beak

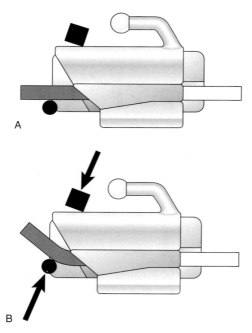

Fig. 17.3 Sealing the space closed at the distal archwire ends. (A) A light wire plier held open, when squeezed partially closed, will turn the annealed end gingivally, precisely at its point of exit from the tube (B).

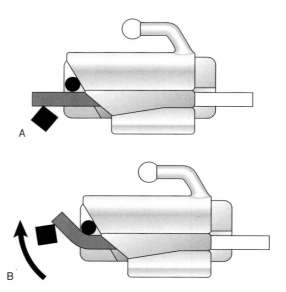

Fig. 17.4 Cinching back to allow a small ingress of space. The fine round beak of a light wire plier preserves a short straight section of distal archwire end (A), whereupon a vertical rotation of the plier, without grasping tightly, turns the remaining distal end gingivally (B).

on the protruding annealed arch end (Fig. 17.3A), a gentle squeeze will seal the space closed (Fig. 17.3B). This can be verified at the midline: it should not be possible to displace the archwire labially.

If, however, no space is available anywhere in the arch, and particularly if there are overlapping contacts, the cinch backs will need to be placed just out of contact with the molar tubes. A small straight section of wire will then remain distal to each tube, which can slide forward through the tube to ease the pressure. Again using a light wire plier, the narrow point of the rounded beak should be placed on the archwire gingivally, against the tube (Fig. 17.4A). This preserves a short straight section, the thickness of the beak, while the square beak rotates the distal end gingivally (Fig. 17.4B). On no account should the plier be squeezed, as this will draw the wire distally through the tube. The amount of slack in the cinch backs can be tested at the front, by the freeplay at the midline.

Whichever type of cinch back is used, the gingival turn-up need never exceed 30 degrees. Bending the wire right up the back of the tube only makes for difficult removal.

Side-Winders and elastomeric modules

Invisible Side-Winders, unlike their predecessors, are fitted first, the modules second. The selection of the correct springs and fitting are as described in Chapter 4. Since Side-Winders are inserted occlusally, their arms will generally point mesially, the main exception being the second premolar in a first premolar extraction case (Fig. 17.5).

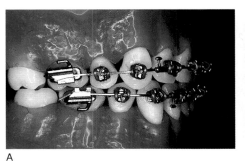
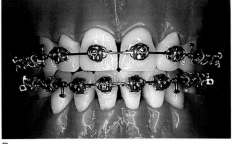
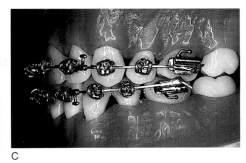

A   B   C

Fig. 17.5 Side-Winder arms point mesially, the main exception being second premolars in a first premolar extraction case.

However, the degree of activation will need to vary according to the tooth and the root movement required. The orthodontist should be aware of this, remembering that a Side-Winder needs to work harder to produce a combination of torque and tip, than tip alone. Incisors are most commonly the teeth requiring both, to which the full activation of Side-Winders, as supplied, is appropriate (Fig. 17.6). This may also apply to lower incisors, where bodily control may be required to boost anchorage, as is commonly practised with straight-wire appliances. On the other hand, with premolars and canines, most of the required correction will be tip, seldom with much torque. Experience with the former Begg appliance demonstrated that simple tip correction could be obtained effectively with appreciably less activation than is provided by an invisible Side-Winder straight from the packet.

Caution is therefore necessary to prevent activation in excess of requirements, particularly to canines and premolars, in which the arc of tip correction lies more along the buccal segment than across the arch. The reciprocal of distal root uprighting is forward crown movement, which represents loss of anchorage. Greater than necessary distal root activation on canines and premolars will therefore encourage a procumbent labial segment. A maximum of 45 degrees of activation between the spring arm and the archwire is quite sufficient (Fig. 17.7). This can easily be achieved by swinging the arm of

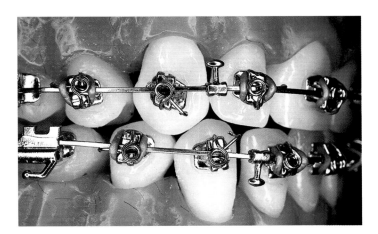

Fig. 17.7 Approximately 45 degrees of activation is generally sufficient on canines, to avoid generating a mesial crown reaction.

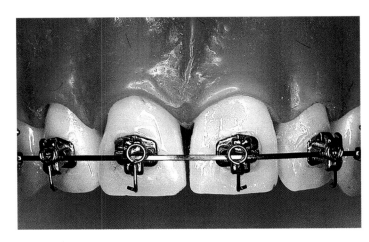

Fig. 17.6 Full activation of Side-Winders is appropriate to incisors requiring torque control.

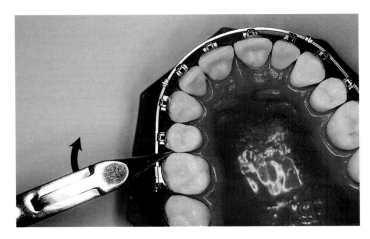

Fig. 17.8 The rotating action of a fine beak plier will deliver an archwire mesially without patient discomfort.

147

the spring gingivally, somewhat past its fitting position, before hooking it on to the archwire.

Placing the modules last, the Straight Shooter needs positive placement to find the bracket, beneath the spring, but practice makes perfect.

Removing the archwires

So long as the archwire ends were thinned and annealed before insertion, removal should be no problem. The cinch backs can be straightened out, with a Howe plier or similar. Because the distal end can never be straightened perfectly, it will not slide forward through the tube freely. The easiest method of removal is to place the tips of a fine beak plier in the embrasure between molar and premolar, while grasping the archwire between the beaks, as close to the molar tube as possible. Rotating the plier forwards (Fig. 17.8), along the long axis of the wire, will 'walk' the wire mesially out of the tube, in three or four movements, without discomfort to the patient.

Stage III checks

Stage III checks

The inspection interval in Stage III is approximately 2 months. As the entire torquing and tip correcting process is essentially built-in, and self-limits automatically, progress and maintenance checks are normally all that is required; it is unusual for an archwire to require removal, except for running repairs.

At each check visit, the following should be observed:

- **Progress of tip and torque.** Both proceed concurrently. Side-Winder springs can be removed selectively as each individual tooth attains its correct torque and tip. However, it should be borne in mind that some relapse of torque and tip is possible, once a spring is withdrawn, particularly if small arch movements are in progress. Active springs should therefore be continued wherever root control needs to be maintained, such as for anchorage purposes. A Tip-Edge bracket can be seen to have self-limited when its upper and lower surfaces lie parallel to the archwire (Fig. 18.1). *Lack of progress is almost invariably due to inadequate mesio-distal space in the arch. It may also be due to incorrect bracket angulation, causing the bracket to self-limit before the desired tip is achieved.*

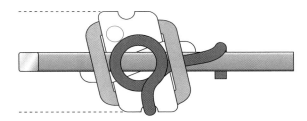

Fig. 18.1 A Tip-Edge bracket has fully expressed when its occlusal and gingival tie wings have become parallel to the rectangular archwire.

- **Available space in the arch.** Except towards the end of root uprighting, it is essential to ensure that up to 1 mm of space exists somewhere in each arch (Fig. 18.2). As explained previously, crowns require additional arch length as they upright, and failure to provide this will stifle the action of the Side-Winders. The procedure for introducing extra wire from the back is described later in this chapter.

Tight or overlapping contacts and rotated incisors (Fig. 18.3) *are sure signs that a limited amount of extra space is needed to make further progress.*

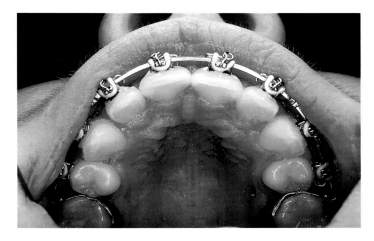

Fig. 18.2 A very small amount of space somewhere in the arch is necessary to allow freedom of uprighting, unimpeded by tight contacts.

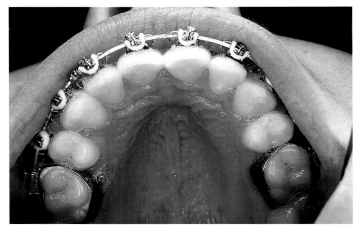

Fig. 18.3 Tight contacts or anterior rotations are indicators of inadequate space during root uprighting.

- **Unwanted space.** More than 1 mm of space is wrong, and should be gathered up by running an elastomeric E-link from crimpable hook to molar hook. At the following visit, the relevant distal arch cinch back will need to be tightened. *Excess space is caused by distal cinch backs that are too slack.*

- **Condition of Side-Winders.** Invisible Side-Winders are seldom lost, as they are retained by the elastic ligatures. However, the loops may become distorted labially, particularly if fiddled with by the patient, and should be bent back to correct shape or replaced. *A labially displaced loop can predispose to escape of the arm lingual to the archwire.*

- **Activation of Side-Winders.** These normally hold their activation without adjustment. However, final torque delivery and apical definition on incisors may require additional activation. 'Hyperactivation' for this purpose will be described opposite.

- **Interarch relationship.** Is the patient regulating the elastic (or headgear) wear adequately to maintain incisor contact, when in the retruded centric position? *The possibility of adverse growth should be considered, but slippage of the interarch relationship almost always identifies a forgetful patient.*

- **The vertical relationship.** Is overbite reduction and buccal segment interdigitation being preserved? *Relapse of overbite in Stage III will most often be the result of inadequate archwire bite sweeps. Vigorous activation of canine Side-Winders can additionally cause overbite increase and infraocclusion of first molars, by reciprocal tipping of the archwire. This should obviously be avoided, but may require 'Class II check' elastics to rectify* (Fig. 18.4).

- **Molar widths.** These will be well controlled by the rectangular archwires. However, in cases where crossbite correction is continuing into Stage III, an archwire may possibly need removal to check width and further adjust, or cancel, molar torque.

- **Second molars.** Towards the end of Stage III, the position and function of second molars will need assessment, with a view to alignment if required. This is outlined in the following chapter.

- **Profile considerations.** This may require confirmation with cephalometric assessment. Is anchorage reinforcement required? *A less than ideal profile may be the result of adverse growth or an inappropriate treatment plan. Too procumbent a profile may also be provoked by excessive activation of Side-Winders, particularly on canines.*

How to admit extra space

This is the most common adjustment needed during Stage III and takes only a few moments to perform. Except when uprighting is almost complete, a very small amount of free space should be available in each arch, to give the crowns the extra 'elbow room' they require as they upright.

First, the four incisors should be released from the archwire by removing the modules. The tapered end of a light wire plier should then be inserted in the contact mesial to the molar band, grasping the archwire immediately mesial to the buccal tube. Gently rotating the handles forward, the action is similar to that described for archwire removal (Fig. 18.5), except that only about half a millimetre of wire will need to be fed through from each side. This needs to be observed carefully. The easiest way to do this is to watch the crimpable

Fig. 18.4 Class II check elastics can be a useful aid in maintaining overbite reduction, or promoting molar occlusion.

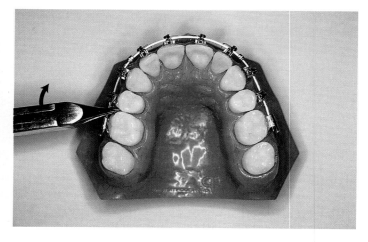

Fig. 18.5 Admitting a small amount of extra space during Stage III, by feeding half a millimetre of wire forward through the molar tube. The incisor ligatures should be removed first.

hook; the slightest forward movement will be sufficient. The elastomeric modules can then be replaced, to gather the incisors fractionally forward. At the start of the third stage, and particularly in extraction cases, it is common to have to repeat this process at consecutive visits.

'Hyperactivation' of Side-Winders

This is only ever required towards the end of treatment on selected teeth, to facilitate the delivery of the final torque prescription, also on those units where ongoing bodily control is required for anchorage purposes. In practice, this means on incisors, almost exclusively. Never should springs be tweaked indiscriminately to speed treatment, particularly down the buccal segments. The outcome would be dragging of anchorage.

Taking a look at the design of a Side-Winder (Fig. 18.6), it will be seen that activation cannot be increased by bending the arm to open up the coils. This is because the leg of the

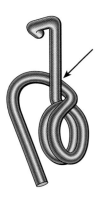

Fig. 18.6 It is not possible to increase Side-Winder activation by unwinding the coils, since the arm will be obstructed by the leg.

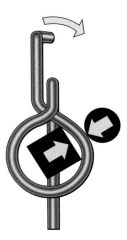

Fig. 18.7 A Side-Winder can be 'hyperactivated' by flattening a small section of the coils with a light wire plier, which effectively expands them (see text).

spring crosses the arm and coils occlusally, to protect them, and therefore prevents the leg from being unwound. Instead, the square beak of a light wire plier should be placed within the coils, the round beak on the outside (Fig. 18.7). A single squeeze will then flatten a small section of the coils, effectively expanding them. Now, the arm actively presses against the leg and would spring past it, if it could. This adjustment can be made without removing the spring. The temptation to do it more than once at a time should be resisted, as excess activation can distort the spring, cause it to unhook or deflect its arm lingually.

Causes of inadequate torque

- **Incorrect bracket.** Use of a bracket designated for a different tooth will obviously express an inappropriate torque value.
- **Misangled bracket.** As with any straight-wire appliance, angling the brackets accurately up the long axis of the tooth is essential to a perfect finish. Angling the jig towards the distal will achieve corrected tip angulation before the bracket has self-limited. The torque will not therefore have been expressed.
- **Incorrect archwire.** Use of an undersized rectangular archwire will reduce torque response; a Side-Winder spring needs the maximum archwire width to produce the torque efficiently.
- **Incorrect bonding position.** Placing a bracket too far incisally or gingivally can significantly alter the final torque angulation.
- **Incomplete bracket engagement.** Even a small rotation will greatly reduce the efficiency of torquing. This may denote tight contact points.
- **Wire ligatures.** Only elastomeric ligatures should be used. Stainless steel ligature ties will not readily adapt their shape to conform to angular changes between archwire and bracket, and will impede uptake of both tip and torque.
- **Tight contact points.** Cinching the archwire ends too tightly will produce tight contact points, denying the crowns the extra space they need when correctly tipped and torqued, as explained previously.
- **Slack Side-Winders.** Seldom a problem, but see 'Hyperactivation' above.
- **Incorrect torque value in archwire.** It is generally better to set the torque in the archwire to over torque slightly, rather than under torque. Obviously, if a retroclined torque value is set in the archwire, this will allow the bracket to self-limit before the desired torque correction has been realized, no matter how active the Side-Winder.
- **Late crown movements.** A Side-Winder will torque a stationary tooth to its intended prescription. If, however, a tooth crown is moved late in the torquing process, there

will be a small delay while the spring torques the root to catch up with its new crown position.

- **Tipped occlusal plane.** It should be remembered that the torque prescription in each bracket is relative to the plane of the archwire. Therefore, if the occlusal plane is allowed to rotate clockwise during treatment (usually due to inappropriate use of Class II intermaxillary elastics or too high elastic forces), a correct torque value achieved between bracket and archwire may appear as under torqued facially.

CASE 10

An adult Class I case with crowding

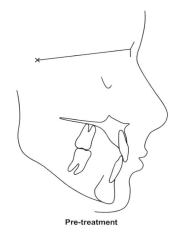

Pre-treatment

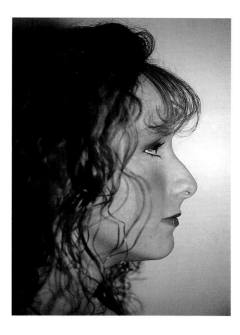

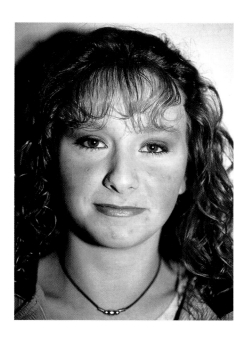

SKELETAL			TEETH		
SNA	°	78.5	Overjet	mm	3.0
SNB	°	76.5	Overbite	mm	4.0
ANB	°	2.5	UI/MxP	°	103.0
SN/MxP	°	12.0	LI/MnP	°	82.0
MxP/MnP	°	28.0	LI-APo	mm	1.5
LAFH/TAFH	%	52.0			

1
At 18 years 3 months, a non-growing adult with a relatively normal skeletal base, retroclined upper incisors and lower incisors just ahead of the A–Po line.

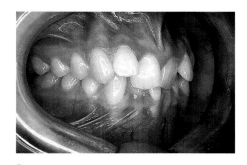

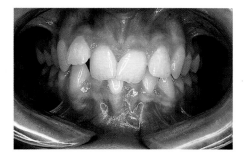

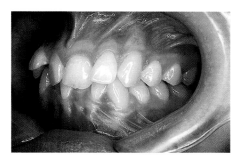

2
Upper and lower incisors are crowded, with some appearance of a Class II division 2 incisor relationship. However, the overbite is only slightly increased, and should not present a treatment problem. Four second premolars are designated for extraction.

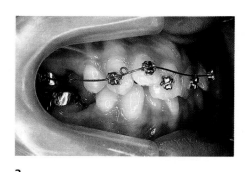
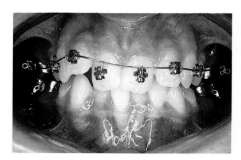
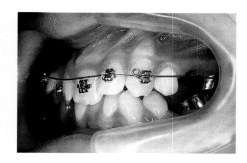

3

Unwanted opening of an adult mandible, which cannot respond with forward growth, should always be borne in mind. However, unlike Case 11, the small amount of bite opening in a near normal skeletal pattern is unlikely to cause posterior extrusion. Normal Tip-Edge Stage I mechanics are therefore appropriate.

Firstly, the retroclined upper central incisors are advanced labially, using a .016 inch high tensile stainless archwire, to which the upper centrals are tied with elastic thread. Light tip-back bends prevent mesial migration of the upper molars.

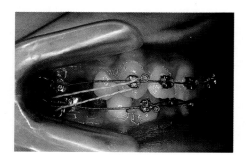
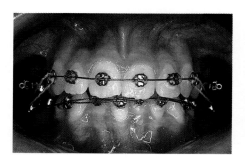
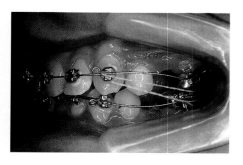

4

Two appointments later, both upper central incisors are fully engaged and clearance is available for lower bonding. Stage I begins, with 50 grams Class II elastics to a .016 inch high-tensile stainless archwire. Moderate anchor bends are placed mesial to all round molar tubes and the premolars are omitted to facilitate overbite reduction. A .012 inch nickel-titanium underarch is engaged to the instanding lower incisors.

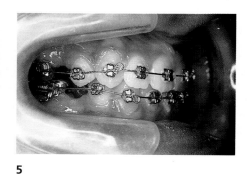
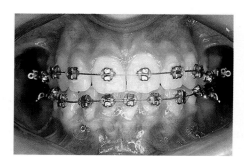
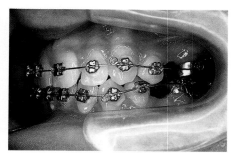

5

Interincisor contact above the lower brackets indicates the end of Stage I. The premolars are bonded for alignment to the rectangular molar tubes, vertical bite sweeps replacing the anchor bends. The round tubes become redundant. Intermaxillary elastics are now only required occasionally, at nights, for the remainder of treatment, to preserve the interarch relationship.

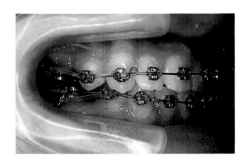
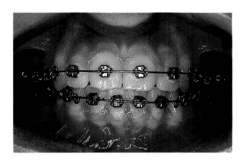
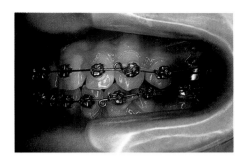

6

Posterior anchorage is predictably stronger in the mature patient and, as anticipated, a considerable amount of extraction space requires to be closed in Stage II.

Swept .020 inch stainless archwires with intra-arch E-6 elastomerics provide space closure. However, the labial segment position appears satisfactory, so that further retroclination is not required. Consequently, brakes are applied in all quadrants (distal root-moving Side-Winders boosting anterior anchorage on first premolars and canines) in order to protract the molars. Note the centreline discrepancy, which requires to be corrected before Stage III.

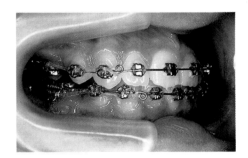
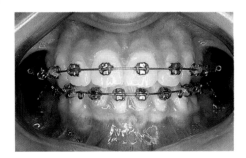
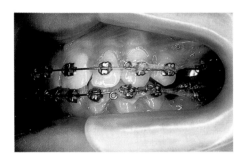

7

No centreline will correct while locked in place by bilateral brakes. Here, towards the end of Stage II, the upper centreline is to the right. Before all extraction space has closed, therefore, the brakes are removed from the upper left canine and first premolar, while continuing the four E-Links. This will allow retraction in the upper left quadrant, protraction elsewhere. The upper centreline will ease across to the left, aided by the brakes remaining in the upper right quadrant.

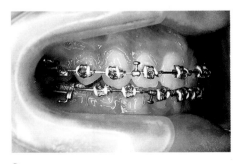
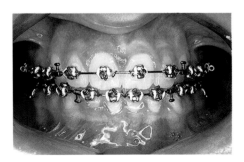
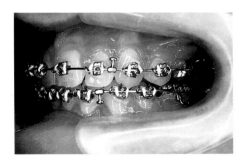

8

With the anterior segment positions well maintained by the brakes, Stage III has relatively little to do, particularly since the previous Side-Winder brakes have eliminated much of the distal crown tip in the canines and premolars. Archwires are .0215 × .028 inch stainless with vertical bite sweeps to retain overbite reduction. Choice of pretorqued archwires results in zero torque in both anterior segments, despite the sweep that would otherwise have caused proclination.

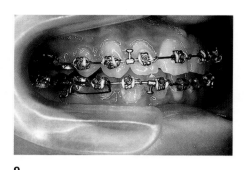
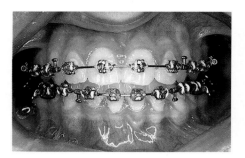
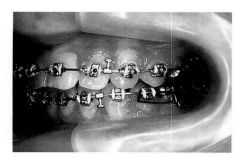

9
Second molars need picking up more frequently in adult patients. Here, Rocke .016 inch sectionals (see Chapter 19) are providing preliminary alignment to the lower second molars, while Stage III nears conclusion elsewhere.

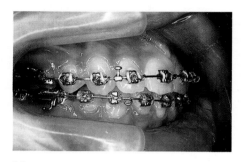
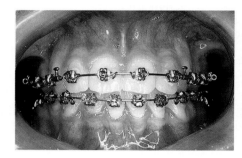
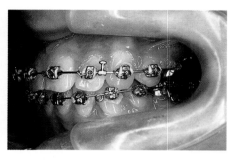

10
Detail alignment of the lower second molars is undertaken at the following adjustment with a .020 inch stainless archwire, converting the first molar tubes to brackets.

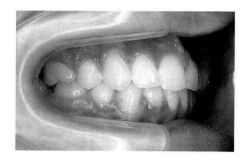
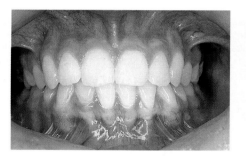
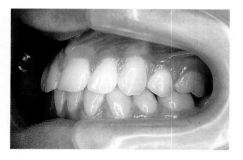

11
Including second molar alignment, Stage III has taken less than 6 months. Each Side-Winder has expressed individually in all three dimensions.

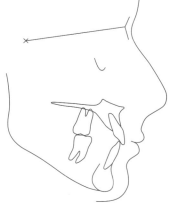

Post treatment

SKELETAL			TEETH		
SNA	°	77.5	Overjet	mm	3.0
SNB	°	76.0	Overbite	mm	2.5
ANB	°	1.5	UI/MxP	°	117.5
SN/MxP	°	12.5	LI/MnP	°	88.5
MxP/MnP	°	26.0	LI-APo	mm	2.0
LAFH/TAFH	%	51.0			

12

The profile has been well preserved.

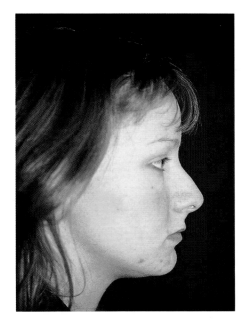

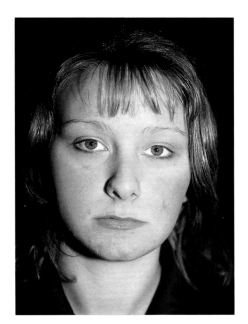

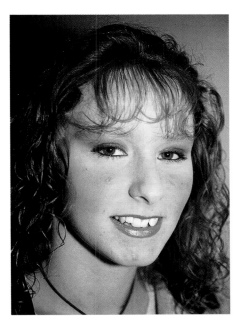

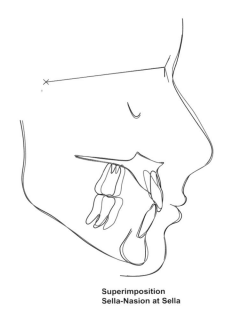

**Superimposition
Sella-Nasion at Sella**

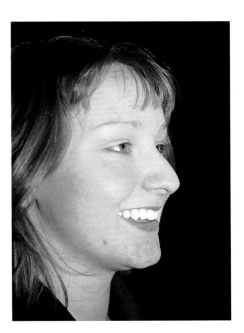

13

The improvement in appearance is largely dental. The upper incisors have been torqued 15 degrees. Note the superimposition of the cephalometric profiles and occlusal plane stability in the non-growing adult.

Treatment time = 1 year 10 months.
Routine adjustments = 13.
Archwires used = 7 (3 upper, 4 lower).
Retention = upper and lower Hawleys, nights only.

CASE 11

An adult Class II division 2 malocclusion with a severe increase in anterior overbite

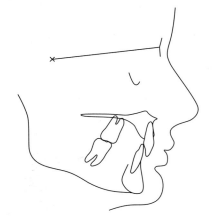

Pre-treatment

SKELETAL			TEETH		
SNA	°	78.5	Overjet	mm	5.5
SNB	°	76.5	Overbite	mm	6.5
ANB	°	1.5	UI/MxP	°	87.5
SN/MxP	°	9.5	LI/MnP	°	92.5
MxP/MnP	°	16.0	LI-APo	mm	-4.5
LAFH/TAFH	%	51.0			

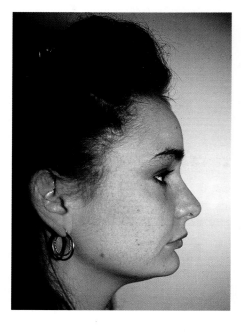

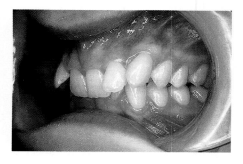

1
A typical Class II division 2 facial type with a low maxillary–mandibular planes angle (16 degrees) and reduced lower face height (51%), at 20 years 7 months. The skeletal base is mild Class II. Predictably, the overbite is greatly increased and complete.

The 'muscular envelope' and bite forces are generally strong in low angle cases, and better able to resist extrusive forces applied to molars. However, with so much overbite reduction required, the risk of provoking unwanted opening of a non-growing mandible, and thereby worsening a Class II tendency, must be considered.

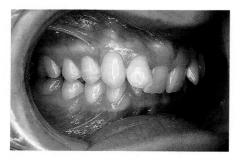

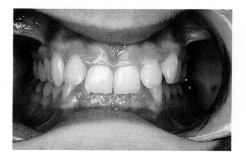

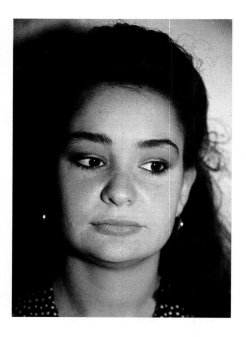

2
The lower incisors are slightly crowded and retroposed on mandibular base (4.5 mm behind A–Po) and will benefit the profile if advanced. The upper laterals are classically proclined and crowded. Both upper buccal segments are forward beyond half a unit Class II.

While this would be a non-extraction case in a growing child, distal driving of upper buccal segments in an adult threatens to be a protracted exercise. The extraction of upper second premolars is therefore preferred, treating to an eventual Class II molar occlusion.

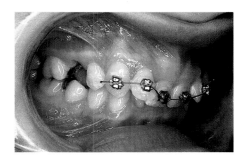
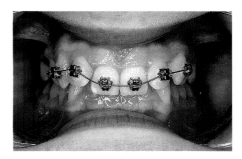
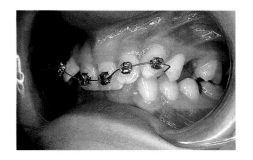

3

As in earlier cases, the upper central incisors are proclined away from the lowers, here using a .016 inch multistrand sectional arch. Mesial drift of the upper molars need not be prevented, so there is no need for a superimposed main archwire at the outset.

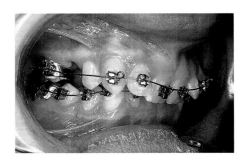
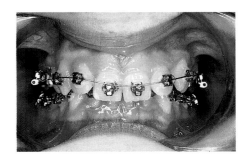
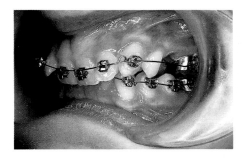

4

One visit later, proclination of the loose tied upper central incisors continues on a .016 inch high tensile stainless archwire with light tip-back bends to the upper molars.

Instead of using lower anchor bends, overbite reduction in the lower arch will be by means of reverse curvature bite sweeps, bonding the premolars from the start and including the second molars early. The risk of molar extrusion and skeletal opening is thereby avoided. This method of overbite reduction is essentially similar to straight wire, except that levelling and inversion of the curve of Spee can proceed irrespective of mesio-distal root angulations. It is therefore quicker and does not require assistance from bite planes.

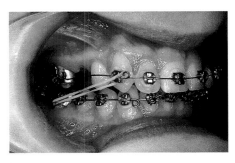
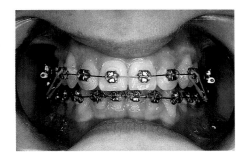
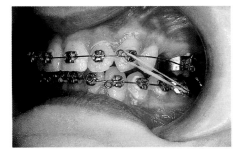

5

The initial .016 nickel-titanium lower archwire is replaced with a .020 inch stainless archwire with a bite sweep. The lower second molars are included. Fifty grams Class II elastics are worn full time to reduce the overjet, while the upper incisors continue to intrude. Experience suggests that upper molars are less liable to extrusion than lower molars, probably due to root configuration. In this case it is significant that the intermaxillary elastics are not being used to lower anchorage bends.

Side-Winders are applied early to the lower incisors, so that torque control can begin as soon as a rectangular wire is fitted.

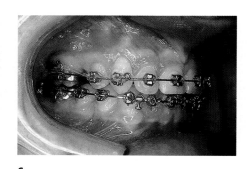
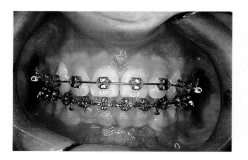
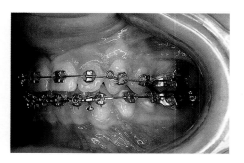

6

Five months later, the bite is open, the overjet is nearly reduced. E-5 elastomerics are closing the upper extraction spaces along a .020 inch stainless archwire with a bite sweep. A lightly swept lower pretorqued .0215 × .028 inch archwire is undercompensated, the sweep not quite cancelling out the 8 degrees of lingual pretorque, in an attempt to build the lower incisor apices as far labially as possible, for ultimate stability.

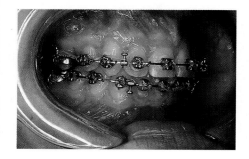
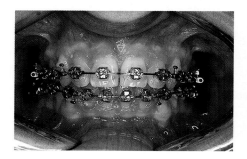
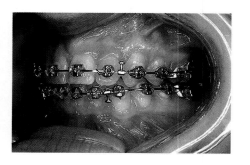

7

In the final phase of Stage III, the upper central incisors have been torqued with Side-Winders against a .0215 × .018 inch stainless wire. A small space is being condensed in the upper right quadrant with a size 4 E-link.

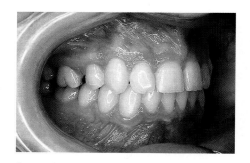
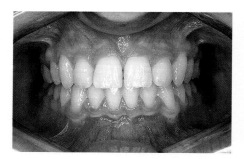
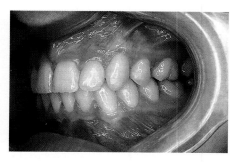

8

At debond, torquing is complete after 5 months in an upper rectangular wire. Overbite reduction has been achieved without the advantage of vertical growth.

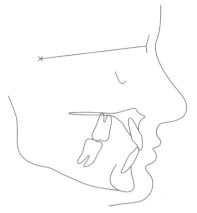

Post treatment

SKELETAL			TEETH		
SNA	°	77.5	Overjet	mm	2.0
SNB	°	76.0	Overbite	mm	1.5
ANB	°	1.5	UI/MxP	°	111.0
SN/MxP	°	10.0	LI/MnP	°	104.0
MxP/MnP	°	16.5	LI-APo	mm	1.0
LAFH/TAFH	%	51.5			

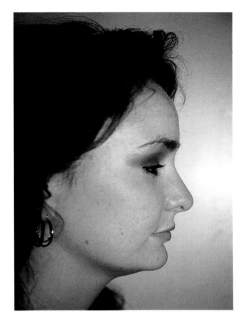

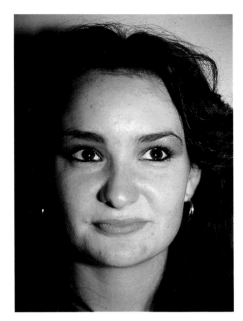

9
The interincisal angle has been overcorrected (128.5 days).

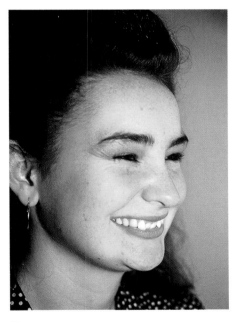

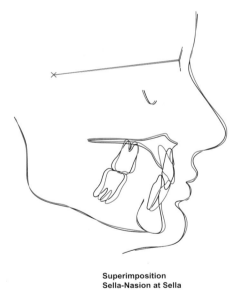

**Superimposition
Sella-Nasion at Sella**

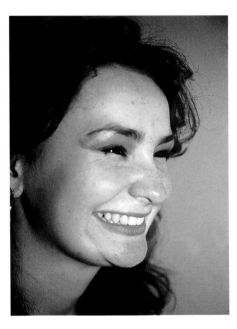

10
Cephalometric superimposition confirms that this degree of overbite reduction has been achieved without skeletal opening and with genuine intrusion of both upper and lower incisors. There is also an improvement in gummy smile.

Treatment time = 1 year 10 months.
Routine adjustments = 14.
Archwires used = 6 (3 upper, 3 lower).
Retention = upper and lower Hawleys, nights only. Lower retention
expected to be long-term.

Precision finishing

Precision finishing

As with any preadjusted appliance, Tip-Edge has an in-built ability to produce a self-limited precision finish. Moreover, in the hands of an experienced operator, it is capable of achieving such goals from considerably more difficult malocclusions than can normally be handled with conventional bracket systems. In this, it is worth stating the obvious, in that the proven intra-arch detail finishing, for which the straight-wire appliance is recognized, is wasted if a Class I interarch relationship cannot be achieved. This happens all too easily if the anchorage demands of the appliance exceed the co-operative abilities of the patient. With a light anchorage technique, this becomes much less likely.

Also, as with any fixed appliance, final detailing depends upon the accuracy with which the case is set up, and it is towards the finish that previously unnoticed small errors in bonding come to light. Of these, incorrect bracket angulations can be corrected surprisingly easily during Stage III, without having to step down into a lighter archwire, so long as the tooth in question has not been allowed to 'over upright'. If it has, the Side-Winder might need reversing for a visit before rebonding.

Assuming correct bracket and tube positioning, all that should be required during the brief finishing phase is occlusal seating; this is essentially the same as with straight-wire appliances. First, however, the second molars should be assessed for inclusion in the appliance.

Picking up second molars

Little has so far been said about second molars. This is because banding of second molars is very seldom required until late in treatment, in marked contrast to conventional appliances. Overbites reduce with only light intrusive forces, since the anterior teeth are not restrained apically, hence the additional vertical 'leverage' afforded by second molars is not necessary. In fact, including second molars from the outset is more often obstructive, adding unwanted friction, particularly during the first and second stages. An exception to this can be seen in Case 11, however, in which reverse curvature bite opening was employed in a deep bite non-extraction adult lower arch.

Routinely, as treatment nears conclusion, the second molars should be assessed carefully for alignment and

function, including testing for non-working side interferences in lateral mandibular excursion. It will be found that lower second molars will require picking up more often than uppers, and most frequently in adults. Conventional straight-wire type .022 × .028 inch second molar rectangular tubes are suitable.

Preliminary alignment can begin in late Stage III by means of a simple sectional device devised by Dr Tom Rocke. While root uprighting is concluding elsewhere with third-stage rectangular archwires, the second molars can be threaded with straight .016 inch high-tensile stainless steel sectionals. These are easily hand bent from a straight length with an annealed distal end. The sectional runs through the channel of the gingival tie wing of the first molar, without being attached to it, and ends mesially with a small occlusally inclined loop. This hooks over the main archwire immediately mesial to the adjacent premolar bracket, and should be squeezed closed for safety (Fig. 19.1). The annealed distal end should be turned lingually for patient comfort. Such a simple sectional will improve alignment and correct mesial crown tip of the second molar, but without disturbing the progress of Stage III elsewhere. Final alignment of the second molars will then entail a full archwire, converting the first molar tubes to brackets in the normal manner.

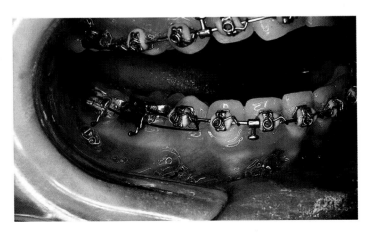

Fig. 19.1 A Rocke section permits initial alignment of second molars while Stage III concludes elsewhere.

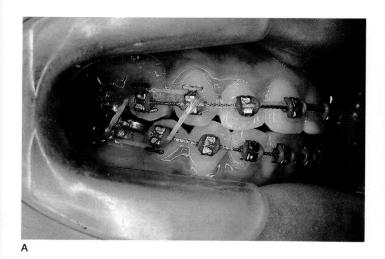
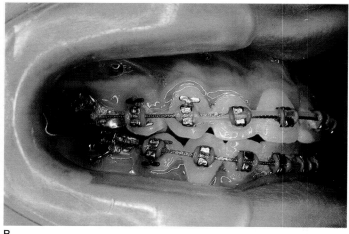

Fig. 19.2 .019 × .025 inch braided archwires and seating elastics (A) promote a tight interdigitation 3 weeks later (B).

The choice of full archwire will depend largely on what is required elsewhere in the arch, as will shortly be outlined. Generally, second molar positioning is a matter of alignment only, for which a flexible round archwire will be appropriate. Rarely, however, a torque discrepancy between first and second molars may be apparent. If so, a rectangular nickel-titanium archwire will be appropriate, rather than an extended rectangular Stage III archwire, which would be too heavy, acting between neighbouring molars.

Occlusal seating

Frequently an accurately set-up case will require no additional archwires beyond Stage III, unless the second molars are included. For a case that does require final seating, vertical elastics can be employed to a combination of molar hooks and gingivally inserted Power Pins, in conjunction with archwires of suitable flexibility. This normally involves no more than the final 3 weeks of treatment, the seating elastics being worn at nights only.

Braided rectangular arches

These are inexpensive, yet effective for small vertical corrections. Archwire size is not critical, but .019 × .025 inch is preferred. If necessary, small vertical offsets can be placed, to aid the vertical elastics in achieving a tight interdigitation. Care should always be taken to ensure strong cinch backs, to prevent space from creeping in: 3 mm of distal projection, annealed, should be bent gingivally, hard against the molar tubes.

Neither Side-Winders nor intermaxillary elastics should be used with multistrand archwires, for obvious reasons, although a short 'rhomboid' elastic configuration, in either a Class II or a Class III direction, can maintain intermaxillary correction (Fig. 19.2).

Titanium-niobium archwires

These may be used in a similar way to braided-wires, but are stiffer. Again .019 × .025 inch is preferred. The extra stiffness can support a lightly active Side-Winder or even light intermaxillary elastics, very briefly. Accurate vertical offsets will be required to facilitate seating, as the wire is too stiff to enable vertical elastics to work unaided. The arch ends should be cinched back hard, without annealing.

Sectioning the main archwire

This is recognized practice with straight-wire, in one or both arches, and can be used with Tip-Edge too.

At the conclusion of Stage III, when all root uprighting is complete, the rectangular archwire can be cut distal to each canine. The premolars and molars will then need tying together with criss-cross ligature wire to the archwire hooks, to prevent spacing (Fig. 19.3). The anterior teeth will also need space prevention, conveniently provided by ligating the canines around the hooks with elastomerics, or running an E-9 elastomeric E-link from canine to canine, as described in Chapter 8. In the absence of an archwire, triangular or rhomboid seating elastics to the buccal teeth need to be somewhat lighter, in order to avoid rotations.

It should be remembered that this method, while easy and apparently effective, preserves least control. In reality, it may be more prone to extrude the buccal cusps into a tight occlusion, producing a convincing final photograph, while leaving the palatal cusps unseated.

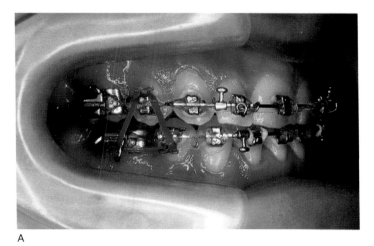
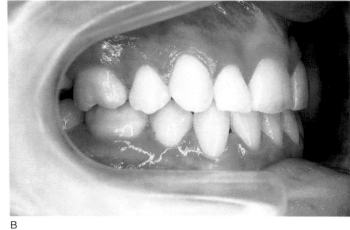

Fig. 19.3 Abbreviation of the upper archwire distal to the canines allows vertical seating of upper buccal segments. The cuspid hooks are laced back to the molars and the anterior units must also be prevented from spacing (A). Night vertical elastics will seat the occlusion in approximately 3 weeks (B).

Crossbite cases

A problem with final 'flexi' arches is lack of arch width control. This should be borne in mind when seating those cases in which the maxillary arch has undergone expansion, because vertical elastics with a flexible archwire will invite contraction of the upper buccal segments. Titanium-niobium will provide more lateral support, but it is sometimes expedient to continue with the stainless Stage III archwire if possible, perhaps finishing the lower arch to the upper in such cases.

Positioners

The tooth positioner is becoming less frequently used in modern orthodontics, due to the improved finishing inherent in preadjusted systems. But it may sometimes avoid the need for finishing archwires, in correctly selected cases, by providing guidance during natural settling. Pre-Fit positioners (Fig. 19.4), which come in a full range of different sizes (for premolar extraction and non-extraction cases), are particularly convenient, but inappropriate where individual tooth size discrepancies exist, such as small upper lateral incisors. A positioner also requires a compliant patient, who can be relied upon to 'exercise' the teeth into it regularly, until longer term retainers can be constructed.

Freedom from immediate laboratory arrangements is the main advantage of the Pre-Fit positioner, allowing a correctly selected patient to be debonded ad hoc, without the need for finishing archwires.

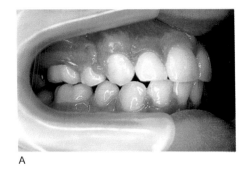
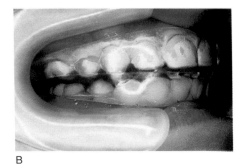
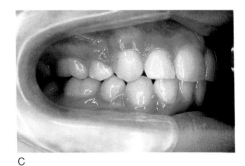

Fig. 19.4 The tooth positioner as a settling aid may take up to 6 weeks.

The non-compliant patient

The non-compliant patient

Like it or not, orthodontic treatment imposes a measure of discipline upon our patients. It is an everyday fact of life that whatever one puts in, is in direct proportion to the gains made in return. And so it is in orthodontics, both with ourselves and with each of our patients. However good the orthodontist, the result that will be achieved, in any case, can be no better than the patient's co-operation allows. Successful orthodontic treatment must be the result of the orthodontist and the patient working together as a team, with mutual understanding and a trust in the capability and efficiency of the process.

Fixed appliances are in some respects the most demanding on patient co-operation, and attempts to produce a 'compliance-free' fixed appliance will inevitably be thwarted by the underlying reliance on the patient for oral hygiene control and prevention of bite damage. However, it obviously behoves the orthodontist to use appliances that are as easy as possible for the patient to use.

In this, Tip-Edge has fundamental advantages. Its initial speed of alignment cannot fail to impress the patient and parent and, being a light force and light anchorage appliance, it can reach its goals with intermaxillary elastics, rather than extraoral forces, for the majority of even the more difficult Class II cases. The bracket itself is smaller and aesthetically superior to twin brackets, adjustment intervals are between 6 and 8 weeks and overall treatment times are generally reduced, dramatically so in major discrepancy situations.

Yet there will always be those patients who are careless or forgetful with their intermaxillary elastics. One ingenious solution to this problem is the use of Outrigger® (TP Orthodontics Inc., La Porte, Indiana, USA) hooks, invented by Dr Christopher Kesling.[1] In carefully assessed cases, these may be strikingly successful in Class II treatment, although they do require to be used with considerable discretion.

Outrigger hooks

These automatically remind the patient to replace the elastics. They do so by the simple method of flicking out sideways, whenever the elastics are not attached. Each Outrigger appliance consists of a pair of hooks, coiled on the end of an interconnecting span, formed from continuous .014 inch

stainless wire (Fig. 20.1). Outriggers are supplied preformed in a range of sizes, according to the desired distance between the hooks, which should be sited distal to the lateral incisor brackets, in lieu of cuspid circles.

Used in Stage I, the base archwire will be .016 inch high tensile stainless steel, as usual, but without cuspid circles. The Outrigger should be threaded on to the archwire from the back, before insertion, taking care to observe the coloured orientation ring, which should be to the patient's right, in order to allow the desired freedom of rotation (Fig. 20.2). The orientation ring can be cut off, once the archwire is fitted. The archwire is placed in the brackets with the Outrigger wire running deep to it, similar to an underarch. Before ligating, the amount of buccal 'spring' in the hooks can be tested, and if necessary adjusted, by altering the curvature of the interconnecting wire, relative to the main archwire as shown (Fig. 20.3). When the elastic is placed, the vertical component of force should rotate the hooks vertically downwards

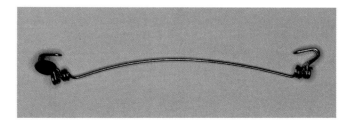

Fig. 20.1 An Outrigger appliance.

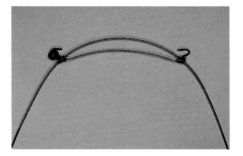

Fig. 20.2 Outrigger threaded on to a .016 inch archwire from the back, with coloured orientation ring to patient's right.

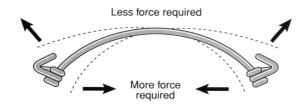

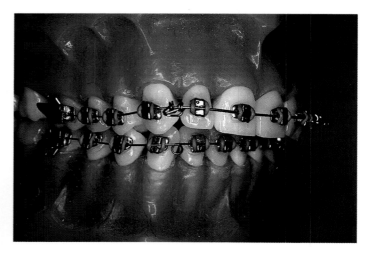

Fig. 20.5 Without the elastics, the hooks flick outwards as a reminder to the patient.

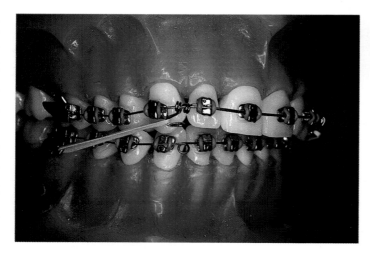

Fig. 20.3 'Tuning' the Outrigger: increasing the curvature increases the flick-out tendency and vice-versa.

Fig. 20.4 With elastics in place, the Outrigger hooks lie vertically. The distal ends of the main archwire are cinched gingivally. This prevents the archwire swinging from side to side and, in a non-extraction case, prevents ingress of spacing.

(Fig. 20.4), without exceeding the light forces (2 ounces or 50 grams) prescribed. To achieve a sufficient vertical component, it is necessary to wear the distal end of each elastic to the molar hook, rather than around the distal archwire end. Whenever the elastic is released, the hook will spring out by up to 90 degrees (Fig. 20.5), causing some inconvenience, but not pain, to the upper lip.

Because cuspid circles are deleted, and the Outrigger hooks must not be impeded by engaging them with elastomerics, an alternative means of preventing the upper anterior teeth from spacing must be used. The simplest method is to run a size 9 E-Link from canine to canine. There is just enough room for this, beneath the archwire and Outrigger assembly. By the same token, the Outriggers do not maintain archwire centralization. This requires the distal arch ends to be cinched gingivally, in order to prevent the archwire from swinging from side to side.

Case selection for Outriggers

One must not make any patient a prisoner to treatment, and Outriggers should be seen as an aid to memory, rather than

any form of compulsion. They are not intended to overcome the problem of the reluctant or rebellious patient, with that look in the eye that forewarns of wrecked appliances. However, they may prove extremely successful, by mutual agreement, in those individuals who mean well but prove to be forgetful. This brings the added bonus of avoiding the need for parental nagging.

Advantages of Outriggers

Quite simply, by ensuring complete elastic compliance, it comes as a revelation, to both orthodontist and patient, as to just how efficiently treatment progresses when intermaxillary elastics are worn literally all the time. Wasted clinical and treatment time is eliminated.

Limitations of Outriggers

- In malocclusions with anterior crowding or excessive incisor spacing, the introduction of the Outriggers will need to wait until the six anterior teeth are approximated and in alignment.
- The patient must carry an adequate supply of spare elastics at all times, for immediate replacement in the event of breakage or loss.
- Part time wear is impossible, yet frequently desirable in Stages II and III. A patient needs to report in at once, in the event of a reversing overjet.
- Use of Outriggers is less easy during Stage II, in extraction cases, as they cannot be used as attachment points for space closing E-Links. Overall condensing elastomerics are less convenient.
- Outriggers are not really suitable for Stage III. The presence of a full thickness rectangular archwire obliges the

Outrigger interconnecting wire to run through the gingival tie wings of the incisor brackets, at some detriment to aesthetics (Fig. 20.6).

- Long term fatigue fracture may occur, which can cause discomfort. Renewal is therefore advised after 3 months in use.

In summary, the Outrigger is more relevant to Stage I than subsequent stages. This is actually less of a disadvantage than might be thought, since it is frequently only the first stage that requires maximum elastic wear; maintenance of the incisor correction during subsequent stages seldom requires more than nightly elastic wear, or evenings and nights, hence placing fewer demands on the patient.

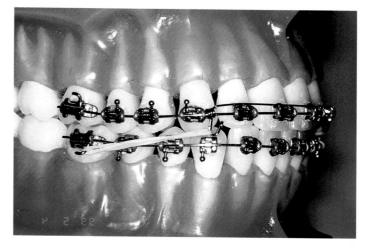

Fig. 20.6 Used with rectangular wire (here shown with conventional brackets) Outrigger hooks become less aesthetic (courtesy of Dr C.K. Kesling).

REFERENCE

1. Kesling CK. A simple means of ensuring Class II elastic wear. Journal of Clinical Orthodontics 2000; 34: 83–87.

Postscript

As modern orthodontics strives increasingly towards perfect finishing, the orthodontist is offered a bewildering plethora of different prescriptions to achieve that end. Without doubt, Andrews' straight-wire appliance, more than any other, has spawned the many variants of Angle's original and brilliant edgewise concept. But with hindsight, might it not be said that fixed appliance technique has concentrated more on the finish than on the journey itself? For without completing the journey, there can be no successful finish. By way of illustration, an aircraft may boast a superb automatic touch-down facility, but this becomes irrelevant if the aircraft itself lacks sufficient range to reach the airport. In clinical terms, this equates to a malocclusion too difficult for an appliance to handle, or beyond the ability or willingness of the patient's co-operation. It is a real world everyday challenge. The increasing reliance of today's orthodontist upon the orthognathic surgeon cannot be ascribed simply to heightened patient awareness.

Certainly, the coming of nickel-titanium and heat-activated archwires has made life easier, both for the orthodontist and the patient, while self-ligating brackets remove some friction from edgewise-derived systems. Yet the modern orthodontist needs to ask a serious question. Why is it still accepted practice to work towards finishing angulations from the moment of first archwire engagement? The answer has to be that the straight wire bracket dictates this. In so doing, by Tip-Edge standards, each tooth becomes an anchorage unit, without choice. As a clinician, Dr Edward Angle himself must have been aware of this, but disbelieved in translation of teeth, in favour of expansion. Also, Angle had no ready means of recovery from tipped angulations. Without doubt, Tip-Edge is here to challenge the established view. Even though it requires a steep new learning curve to depart from convention, the results surely expand the horizons of fixed appliance capability.

To conclude with the aircraft analogy, wheels are not required during flight. They fold away to make the journey easier, but become vitally necessary when landing. If taking up finishing angulations early in treatment makes the journey more difficult, the philosophy behind Tip-Edge makes obvious sense. Finishing angulations, by their very definition, do not become necessary until the finish of treatment.

In the future: 'Tip-Edge Plus'

At the time of writing, a modified version of the Rx-1 Tip-Edge bracket is about to be launched by TP Orthodontics, Inc. known as 'Tip-Edge Plus'. The aim of the new bracket is to achieve Stage III root movements by means of a heat activated nickel-titanium auxiliary archwire, thereby eliminating the need for Side-Winders.

The Tip-Edge Plus bracket looks the same as the standard Rx-1 bracket, and has identical slot dimensions and geometry (see Fig. A). However, in addition to the vertical slot for auxiliary springs, each bracket carries a horizontal slot for the auxiliary archwire, known as the 'deep tunnel'. This runs almost at right angles to the vertical slot (thereby forming a hidden 'Plus' sign within the bracket)(see Fig. B). Since the vertical slot and the deep tunnel cross, they cannot be used simultaneously. The deep tunnel is not accessible from the labial and can only be threaded, so that accidental disengagement of the auxiliary archwire is impossible, and rotational control is boosted.

In essence, Tip-Edge Plus stays faithful to all the Tip-Edge concepts, as described in this book. Stages I and II are carried out identically, including the use of Side-Winders for braking, Power Tipping and centreline correction. However, while Stage III with rectangular archwires remains the same in principle, the uprighting forces are generated by the small diameter auxiliary archwires in the deep tunnels, concealed beneath the rectangular archwires. On incisors, the deep tunnels are angled slightly, to promote closer final approximation between the bracket and the upper and lower surfaces of the rectangular archwire.

The potential advantages of a 'spring-free' Stage III are improved aesthetics, oral hygiene and patient comfort. It also avoids incorrect selection and accidental detachment of springs. Allthough initial clinical trials show considerable promise, it remains to be seen how the spring return properties of a 'thermo ni-ti' underarch compare with individual stainless steel springs, in achieving a precise torque and tip outcome. Meanwhile, Side-Winders are proven. They allow variation in activation between canines and incisors and have 'power in reserve' right up to the finishing point, to ensure complete correction, as well as maintaining subsequent bodily control.

Tip-Edge Plus is an attractive concept which may well become the future for differential tooth movement. At the present time, however, it requires extensive clinical experience to gain full endorsement.

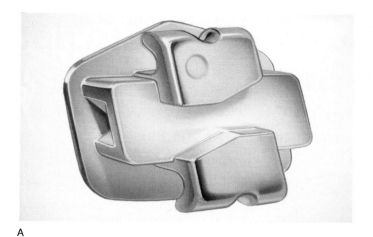

A

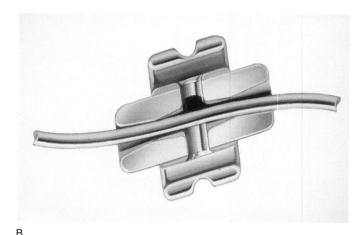

B

Fig. (A) A Tip-Edge Plus bracket (maxillary right canine) is similar in dimension and appearance to the standard Rx-1 bracket. The bevelled exit of the deep tunnel can be seen deep to the main archwire slot. (B) A Tip-Edge Plus bracket (maxillary right canine) seen from the lingual, without its mesh pad. The vertical deflection of the deep tunnel auxillary wire will generate distal root tip in lieu of a Side-Winder spring. The rectangular main archwire is omitted from the illustration.

TIP-EDGE TREATMENT SEQUENCE

Stage	Functions	Archwires	Technique	Adjustment interval
Tip-Edge treatment sequence				
1	Alignment of upper and lower anterior segments Closure of anterior spaces Correction of increased overjet or reverse overjet Correction of increased overbite or anterior open bite Buccal segment crossbite correction	.016 inch high tensile stainless .014 inch nickel-titanium underarches to align instanding anteriors	Omit premolars if overbite increased (in which case use round molar tubes) Intermaxillary elastics and anchor bends as required E9 E-link to close anterior spacing Ligate canine brackets to cuspid circles once anteriors aligned	6 weeks
End of Stage I	Bond premolars if initially excluded (increased overbite cases only) and align to rectangular molar tubes	Continued .016 inch high-tensile stainless	Remove anchor bends and wipe in vertical bite sweeps Replace archwires in rectangular molar tubes Continue canine to cuspid circle ligation until Stage II Continue traction as necessary to maintain incisor contact	3 weeks
II	Closure of residual spacing, by retraction or by protraction Correct centrelines Continuing crossbite correction Maintain Stage I corrections	.020 inch high tensile stainless (option of .022 inch in first molar extraction or crossbite correction cases)	Rectangular tubes. Bite sweeps if required Horizontal E-links for space closure Brakes, if protraction necessary Unilateral brakes for centreline correction Continue traction as necessary to maintain incisor contact	6 weeks
End of Stage II	Derotation of first molars Levelling of first molars if necessary	Same	Offsets and toe-ins to first molars following space closure Consider anti-tip bends to seat distal first molar cusps	3 weeks
III	Correction of torque and tip angles Attainment of optimal facial profile Maintain Class I occlusion	.0215 × .028 inch stainless (for choice of plain or pretorqued, see Chapter 16)	(Cephalometric X-ray first) Rectangular molar tubes; crimp-on hooks; invisible Side-Winders Consider anterior torque modification in Class III cases (see Chapter 16) Continue traction as necessary to maintain Class I occlusion	2 months
End of Stage III	Assess need to include second molars Final detailing, seating, etc	.016 inch sectional Rocke sectionals ? free the buccal segments from main archwire ? .019 × .025 inch braided ? .019 × .025 inch titanium-niobium	For preliminary alignment of second molars to first molars Vertical seating elastics, nightly, to Power Pins and/or molar hooks (Consider Pre-Fit positioner) (see Chapter 19)	3 weeks

Further reading

Cronin T. Arch wire sequencing in Tip-Edge treatment. Journal of General Orthodontics 2001; 12: 31–33.

Harrison JE. Early experiences with the Tip-Edge appliance. British Journal of Orthodontics 1998; 25: 1–9.

Kesling CK. Improving incisor torque control with nickel titanium torque bars. Journal of Clinical Orthodontics 1999; 33: 224–230.

Kesling CK. Case report: Tip-Edge treatment of a Class II division I malocclusion with an anterior open bite. Journal of General Orthodontics 1992; 3: 19–22.

Kesling PC. Tip-Edge Guide and the Differential Straight-Arch technique, 4th edn. Two Swan Advertising; 2000.

Kesling PC, Rocke RT, Kesling CK. Tip-Edge brackets and the Differential Straight-Arch technique. In: Graber TM, Vanarsdall RL, eds. Orthodontics current principles and techniques. St Louis: CV Mosby; 2000.

Kift RJ. Non-extraction Tip-Edge appliance management of a moderate Angle Class II division 1 malocclusion commenced in the late mixed dentition. Australian Orthodontic Journal 2001; 17: 47–54.

Knight H. The effects of three methods of orthodontic appliance therapy on some commonly used cephalometric angular variables. American Journal of Orthodontics and Dentofacial Orthopaedics 1998; 93: 237–244.

Lawson R, Durning P. Use of Tip-Edge brackets in patients with repaired alveolar clefts. Journal of Clinical Orthodontics 1998; 32: 84–88.

Miyajima K, Iizuka T. Treatment mechanics in Class III open bite malocclusion with Tip-Edge technique. American Journal of Orthodontics and Dentofacial Orthopaedics 1996; 110: 1–7.

Morein S. Tip-Edge challenges older appliances. Journal of General Orthodontics 1996; 7: 6–11.

Pancherz H, Loffler A, Obijou C. Efficiency of root torquing auxiliaries. Clinical Orthodontic Research 2001; 4: 28–34.

Parkhouse RC. Differential tooth movement in 'uphill' cases. American Journal of Orthodontics and Dentofacial Orthopaedics 1992; 101: 491–500.

Rocke RT. Employing Tip-Edge brackets on canines to simplify straight-wire mechanics. American Journal of Orthodontics and Dentofacial Orthopaedics 1994; 106: 341–350.

Index